OUR LOST CHILDREN

SILENT VOICES – DAMAGED LIVES

Sue Wood

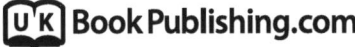

Design, typesetting and publishing by UK Book Publishing

www.ukbookpublishing.com

ISBN: 978-1-916572-86-7

I dedicate this book to all of the many charities which work with children and young people in the UK. Many of them are mentioned in the following pages and the work they do is life-changing.

*

All royalties from the sale of this book will be donated to the charity 'Together for Short Lives'. Together for Short Lives' purpose is to ensure that every seriously ill child, and their family, has high quality children's palliative and end of life care, when and where they need it.

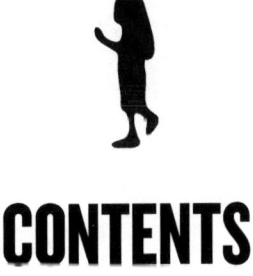

CONTENTS

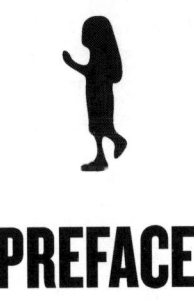

PREFACE

I have written three books which record the actions of the Conservative government from 2019 to 2023. They are called '**Beneath the Bluster,' Behind the Headlines'** and **'Britain Betrayed'.** The first two cover the premiership of Boris Johnson and the last one covers the premiership of Liz Truss and the first ten months of Rishi Sunak.

When I am asked why I write these books I say it is because of a sense of burning anger. Burning anger at the incompetence and the cavalier attitude of this government, but specifically burning anger at the way this government has treated and continues to treat our children and young people.

I have written a lot about children in my previous books and I had intended to leave it at that, but two instances recently made me want to write again.

A tiny paragraph tucked away on a page in the *Times* by Tom Saunders on 28th September 2023 says that children's suffering during the pandemic was preventable. The Children's Rights Organisation says that the closure of schools and playgrounds had "long lasting and era-defining impacts." 'Save the Children' have written a report called "What About the Children?" and the principal finding of the report is that the "worst impacts of the pandemic for children could have been prevented **if their voices were heard** and if children's rights were considered by UK decision-makers." Their written evidence will be submitted to the Covid Inquiry this month (September 2023) but it would appear to be a fact that the loss of learning, child abuse and worsening mental health problems could have been avoided.

Then a Primary Head Teacher speaking to my niece yesterday (27th September) said: "Children are at the bottom of the list and were all through the pandemic and since. This lot don't care," which is a complete endorsement of what I have always said.

But "**if their voices were heard**" is the phrase that stands out for me and this is why I am writing this book. I will make their voices heard loudly and clearly in the following pages.

******

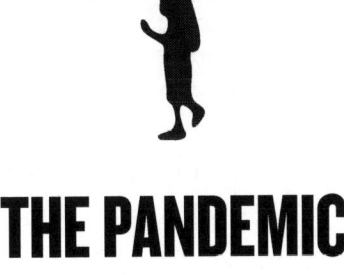

THE PANDEMIC

I am absolutely amazed that this report, has not been given wider coverage in the media. It is really important and some of its conclusions need to be addressed now. Written on behalf of the Children's Rights Organisations, a group established for the UK Covid-19 Inquiry incorporating 'Save the Children', 'Just for Kids Law' and the 'Children's Rights Alliance for England', it makes very disturbing reading. It is **not** saying that lockdowns were unnecessary but it **is** saying that children's needs and requirements were different from those of adults and this should have been accounted for.

I have just read the entire report and it is interesting to note that they had feedback and discussions with the Youth Advisory Board at 'Save the Children'. This is a group of 12-18-year-olds who agreed to share their experiences with them. **So their voices are here, all the way through the report**.

As they say, I think we all found the messaging confusing but for children and teenagers it was especially so. This caused unnecessary stress, uncertainty and feelings of immense responsibility for them.

As the report notes: "Children have rights enshrined in UK and international law including the right to an education, the right to play, and the right to live free from harm, abuse and neglect. They also have the right to be heard. These rights were not sufficiently considered by decision-makers over the two years of pandemic policy making."

They go on to say: "The valiant efforts of experts and campaigners ensured that children received some protection, but their advice was too often ignored. If it was clear to footballer Marcus Rashford that more support was needed to prevent children going hungry, there is no justification why decision-makers were not aware of this. We are yet to discover the full impact of pandemic policies on children. At every stage there are concerns, from language and cognitive development in the early years to academic progress for school pupils and the mental wellbeing of teenagers. But there is hope. If action is taken now and plans are put in place for future pandemics, recovery is possible."

Anne Longfield, England's former Children's Commissioner, said ministers were indifferent to children during lockdown.

Children will be living in the "long shadow" of the pandemic for the next two decades thanks to the government's "indifference" to them during lockdown, she told the Covid inquiry.

"The devastating impact [of lockdown] on certain groups of children was clearly predictable."

Then there are children and young people who are especially vulnerable.

"Many of the decisions taken during the pandemic made an assumption that children live at home with their parents. But this is not the case for some children in the social care system and the criminal justice system. Pandemic policies did not consider the unique circumstances of these vulnerable groups of children, in some cases leading to extreme trauma. Children went long periods without face-to-face contact with loved ones and trusted support workers. It is our view that the most vulnerable children in society who don't live at home – including those in custody and care – were entirely forgotten by policy-makers during the pandemic."

She said she tried repeatedly to talk to the government about the impact their pandemic policies were having on children.

"It was very clear that there was no one at the cabinet table who was taking responsibility for children's best interests," she said. "I was always told it was the role of the Secretary of State for Education but it was very clear he wasn't part of some of those discussions. There was an empty chair at the table."

She criticised the government for not making more effort to get vulnerable children back into schools when restrictions on attendance were partially lifted. For a long time, she said, only about 4% of vulnerable children attended school. That later rose to between 10% and 12%.

This report is divided into three categories: Education, Play and Socialisation, and Safety.

EDUCATION

We all know that the promises by the government of computers in every household for remote learning was not accomplished and as the report says, "At first, the government was slow to address the unequal experiences of remote learning – almost a year into the pandemic, only one in five schools were able to supply laptops and tablets to all pupils who needed one."

'Barnardo's' chief executive Javed Khan said in January 2021 that "urgent action" was needed to make internet access more affordable.

Disadvantaged families are being "locked out" of education as they cannot afford the costs of online learning, and Ofcom said 6% of UK families struggled with broadband costs, while 5% could not afford their mobile bills.

It was up to many charities to encourage organisations to donate computers when they could.

Although by March 2021, 1.3 million laptops, tablets and routers had been despatched by the government there were still many families who had little or no access to the internet, or who simply could not afford it.

Katie Schmuecker, from the 'Joseph Rowntree Foundation,' said: "For people in poverty, high costs and low incomes can mean internet access is out of reach, or incredibly expensive when accessed through pay-as-you-go [mobile data] tariffs. This leaves children locked out of an education."

The report recommendations are that schools and early years' settings should be classified as essential infrastructure for future health emergencies. The decision to close schools cannot be made by ministers alone and should be considered only as a last resort.

Our schools were closed for longer than anywhere else apart from Italy. Our children lost twice as many learning days as in France, Hungary, Spain and Austria and the Swedes never closed schools at all.

We remember the time when Gavin Williamson opened some schools on June 1st 2020 only to close them again on June 9th just a few days later causing parents and children further stress.

Again on January 4th 2021 the PM (Johnson) said yes schools will open for the spring term tomorrow (the 5th) as planned and then at 8pm (on the 4th) were told that no actually they would be closed. Many young children went to bed thinking they would be going to school in the morning, only to wake up to find that they were not. Absolute incompetence.

Further recommendations are that they need to "provide the full £13.5bn of educational recovery funding that is needed directly to schools and colleges, giving them autonomy in how funds are spent to ensure students are encouraged to come back to school and fulfil their potential."

And then there was complete fiasco over the public exams of A level and GCSEs in the summer of 2020.

Due to the covid-19 pandemic, students could not take their final exams, and instead, computer modelling was used to assign grades. Pupils taking GCSEs and A-levels in England were told that would have their grades awarded by a combination of teacher assessment, class ranking and the past performance of their schools.

Ofqual began to lay out details of the new system, but experts quickly became worried that relying on teacher assessments was likely to penalise students from disadvantaged backgrounds.

In England, they were given grades by the official exam regulator, Ofqual.

Teachers were asked to supply for each pupil for every subject:

- An estimated grade

- A ranking compared with every other pupil at the school within that same estimated grade

These were put through an algorithm, which also factored in the school's performances in each subject over the previous three years.

Well this did not go very well at all.

When results were unveiled, there was shock and anger at what looked like clear injustices. The algorithm used to determine grades was widely criticized for being unfair and biased. There was uproar after about 40% of A-level results were downgraded by Ofqual, which used the formula based on schools' prior grades.

The government faced immense pressure to explain itself, and ministers went silent before the Education Secretary emerged to announce a major U-turn. Students who had been downgraded could now use the grades their schools had predicted.

Now who was the Education Secretary again? Oh yes how could we forget? Gavin Williamson had to turn out and acknowledge "significant inconsistencies" in the grading process and apologise for the "distress" caused.

He also announced that GCSE results would be decided according to teacher assessments.

It is interesting to note that Roger Taylor, Ofqual's Chair, revealed that Ofqual told the government in March that awarding grades using a statistical model was "the worst-case scenario".

"At the outset, our initial advice to the Secretary of State was that the best way to handle this was to try to hold exams in a socially distanced manner, and that our second option was to delay exams. But the third option, if neither of these was acceptable, was to have to try and have some form of calculated grades," Mr. Taylor said.

"It was the Secretary of State who then subsequently took the decision and announced – without further consultation with Ofqual – that exams were to be cancelled and a system of calculated grades was to be implemented."

Ofqual's senior leadership told MPs that Ofqual should not be blamed for the fiasco that engulfed this summer's exams in England, and accused the Education Secretary, of causing the weekend of chaos that followed the publication of A-level results.

Those poor children. No-one was listening to sensible advice and they had Gavin Williamson in charge.

Just to remind you that Gavin Williamson was sacked by Theresa May, then appointed a minister by Boris Johnson and then sacked by Johnson and then appointed again by Rishi Sunak and then resigned before he was pushed in November 2022.

****

Then with much of the focus being on schools, we mustn't forget UK University students who reported feeling forgotten by the government, with no rebates offered on tuition fees and calls growing for rent refunds as many students were asked not to return to campuses during the pandemic.

Many of them spoke about how the pandemic impacted on their mental health.

Let us listen to them now.

"There's a real emphasis on schoolchildren at the moment, and I understand it's hard on everyone, but they aren't away from their families. They get to go home to their mum and dad and have that support. When you're at uni, you're on your own."

"My mental health was at 'the lowest it's ever been' during the first term."

"Last week, Boris Johnson didn't address us in the press conference announcing the national lockdown in England at all. It shows he doesn't really have any care or concern, especially for our mental health."

"What I'm concerned about now, and a lot of my peers feel the same, is that we've all got exams coming up in January, and we're all feeling broken and defeated,"

"Gavin Williamson cancelled A-levels and GCSEs, but there was no mention of our exams in a few weeks."

"I have had numerous friends express their own increasing difficulties with depression and anxiety."

"One housemate has been breaking public health rules to make regular trips to nearby cities, attend parties and have visitors over. When I once

spoke to her about going to one of these parties, she didn't see the problem, saying that she left before the police turned up."

"She also had one of her friends spend the weekend at ours, which I first found out when I found a stranger in our kitchen."

"I had people I spoke to in my classes, but outside of my classes, I would spend time sitting in the car or sitting in the toilets, waiting for any free time to be over,"

"I had friends who graduated last year, and they still haven't heard anything about their graduation."

The overwhelming impression is one of intense loneliness and a feeling of being abandoned.

****

PLAY AND SOCIALISATION

Children desperately need to get outside to meet friends and to play. Teenagers too, need to socialize and have fun.

But this report notes that, "Even after one week of lockdown, experts were urging the government to support children's play to help them and their parents cope, and multiple campaigns over 18 months urged the government to clarify the guidance and let children play outdoors. Pandemic policies unnecessarily harmed children and young people's social development and mental health because decision-makers did not consider the impact of the rules on children."

The government made no allowances for children whatsoever.

"Police guidance on what constituted a "reasonable excuse" to leave home during lockdown gave specific examples of adult exercise such as running and yoga but did not mention children or play.

Grassroots sports clubs and other spaces for children's activity remained closed whilst pubs, restaurants and even schools reopened. Playground closures disproportionately affected children in poverty and marginalised communities who are less likely to have access to a private outdoor space"

And then "from 13 May 2020, adults were allowed to exercise outdoors but there was no change to the rules regarding playgrounds."

The blinkered thinking was very damaging.

"Young people reported that the public and police interpreted trips to the park, and teenagers meeting up, as violations of lockdowns, and young people from racial minorities were more likely to receive fines in the first lockdown."

Then the most disgusting phrase was used by this government and I remember being shocked by it. Everyone knew that children were less likely to spread the virus of Covid but the "**Don't Kill Granny**" campaign was deliberately targeted at young children and was extremely upsetting and unnecessary. They were being told not to hug their grand-parents in case they gave them Covid.

The report goes on to note that:-

"The 1:1 rule in England allowed adults to meet a friend outside but prevented younger children from doing the same. Even in the third national lockdown in 2021, when children aged 0-5 were exempted from the rule, children aged 5 – 12 who required adult supervision were left out.

"Rule of Six" included children, which meant six individual adults from six different households could meet, but two-parent families each with two children could not.

Support bubbles were not in place for families during the first lockdown, meaning grandparents could not support with childcare and separated families could not see each other.

Then in June 2020, 100+ leading psychologists wrote an open letter to Gavin Williamson (yes I know) and said, "As experts working across disciplines, we are united as we urge you to reconsider your decision and to release children and young people from lockdown."

But nothing was done.

They recommended the following for the future:-

* Develop a National Play Strategy that prioritises children's free outdoor play, including a duty for local authorities to ensure sufficient provision for play in the community and ensure play is included in a ministerial portfolio.

* Properly fund a Children's Recovery Plan to tackle the long-term effects on children's social and emotional development and educational attainment caused by Covid-19 pandemic and lockdowns.

****

SAFETY

Again we all know about the dangers children can face whilst browsing on computers and here we are encouraging all children to access computers for remote home learning.

"The lack of infrastructure and support for children during the pandemic meant it was harder to identify children at risk at a time when they were spending much more time on their devices and social media. Perpetrators took advantage of this, finding new ways to contact children during lockdown, creating 'the perfect storm' in terms of children's online safety. Child criminal exploitation also increased further during the pandemic as children were more vulnerable out of school, receiving less contact with social services, and organised crime gangs moved to online forms of grooming and recruitment."

Their recommendations here are:-

- Hold technology companies to account for safety of children on their sites, provide a robust regulatory framework and create a child safety advocate to fight for children at risk of online harm.

- Test future pandemic policy guidance with children and parents and create child- and youth-friendly information about accessing health services and staying safe that is accessible and relevant.

****

This is a much needed report. I am quite sure that some will say 'well it's all very well with the benefit of hindsight' but I say there is no excuse for children to be ignored in this way. Those who choose to govern should be aware of the needs of children. It just needs some intelligence, compassion, knowledge and an ability to listen to children themselves. Over 100 people professionally involved with children's well-being wrote to the government but were ignored.

This is why the report's final recommendations are so important. I pick out just a few.

They write that in order to protect children's interests in governance and policy-making we need to:-

- Appoint a Cabinet Minister for Children with cross-departmental responsibility for driving forward implementation of a Child Rights Action Plan.

- Enshrine children's rights into UK law by incorporating the UN Convention on the Rights of the Child (UNCRC) in full, making

Child's Rights Impact Assessments a statutory requirement for all new legislation.

- Publish a National Recovery Plan for children, young people and families which addresses issues outside of education and a National Play Strategy.

- Urgently publish a children and young people's Mental Health Plan that will address long waiting lists for services and place more emphasis on early intervention as well as prevention and ensure this is backed up with adequate and sustainable investment

- Set out a comprehensive, long-term funding settlement for children's services that invests at least £2 billion a year in early intervention and therapeutic services.

- Invest £2.6bn, as an absolute minimum, in children's social care targeted specifically at deprived areas.

- Develop a national strategy and improvement plan to address racial disproportionality and repair the harms to children who were in prison during Covid-19, alongside a plan with clear timescales for closing children's prisons.

This report argues that there are some universal truths which must be recognised:-

1. The UK's pandemic policies harmed children and young people.

2. Their rights and interests were not adequately considered by decision-makers. We must take action now to prevent a generation of children and young people being defined forever by their experience of the Covid-19 pandemic.

And just before I leave this chapter I need to understand this. We have just seen a programme called 'Partygate' on the BBC. This depicted the parties held in No 10 Downing Street during lockdown. It didn't tell us anything we didn't already know but it brought home just how disgusting it all was. So many people cheek-by-jowl dancing, singing, drinking, vomiting, spilling wine and at least one couple having sexual intercourse which brings the lack of social distancing to a new high. For this Boris Johnson was found to have broken lockdown rules and was fined £50.

And then also during lockdown, an 18 year old student organised a snowball fight out in the open snowy spaces of Yorkshire where children were running away from each other to avoid being hit by a snowball and were enjoying the wonderful fresh air. For this he was fined £10,000. **My question is, why such disparity?**

And just today (31st October 2023) we hear from the Covid inquiry that the then Education Minister Gavin Williamson ignored Covid safety concerns from the unions about children in schools needing to wear masks for fear of looking weak by giving in to the unions.

So he risked the lives of children in order to make a political point.

****

THE PRIVILEGED ELITE

There are still more unedifying exposures coming from the Covid inquiry. Today (November 1st) Helen MacNamara took the stage and painted a picture of excessive bullying and misogyny in cabinet discussions. She was deputy Cabinet Secretary from 2020 to 2021 and explained how the needs of children and women were completely ignored during that time. She said that **"the exclusion of a female perspective led to significant negative consequences".** She said that because the backgrounds of senior people in government were very comfortable it gave them a "narrow perspective" on the problems facing Britain. In other words they had no idea what it was like to be in a two bedroom flat with no garden in a family of four or what it was like to cope as a single mother or to be a woman suffering from domestic abuse. There were very few women giving views and when they were, they were talked over by the men who only wanted to talk about football. As she said "There wasn't enough thinking about the overall experience of children who might not have quite the same privilege as the people in the rooms of Whitehall taking decisions." They took very little account of how decisions such as closing schools would affect mothers. Issues such as child care and carers were completely neglected and never even considered.

Every single day of the Covid Inquiry confirms the fact that we were governed by people totally unsuited for the job. Number 10 was a complete circus of inadequacy, chaos and incompetence. And the indifference to the suffering of children was on an unprecedented scale.

****

"There can be no keener revelation
of a society's soul than the way
in which it treats its children."

Nelson Mandela

****

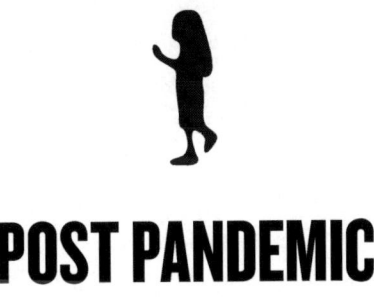

POST PANDEMIC

Well, eventually the pandemic was over but the suffering goes on.

As we have seen, all children need safe environments where they can go to meet friends, to play sport or to take part in fun, new activities.

But for years now schools have been selling off their sports fields, and youth clubs have been closing due to lack of funds. And of course, since the pandemic, things have got a lot worse. Swimming pools are also now facing higher energy costs and having closed during lockdown are struggling to re-open or are closing permanently. This is obviously having a directly negative impact on the health of our children.

All youth clubs were forced to temporarily close as part of coronavirus lockdown measures announced in the UK back in March 2020.

They were free to re-open on 29 June 2021 but with major social distancing restrictions in place, including the number of people allowed in venues at any one time. However the 'National Youth Agency' said 2,000 of the 10,000 youth projects in England will struggle to re-open following the loosening of Covid-19 restrictions and a leading educational charity has warned that thousands of youth centres across England could close permanently.

Research shows that England faces a wholesale closure of youth organisations, leaving a generation of vulnerable young people without life-changing support.

In 2021 almost two-thirds of youth organisations with incomes under £250,000 said they were at risk of closure, with 31% saying they might have to shut in the next six months.

In January 2021 Anna Alcock, the head of engagement and advocacy at 'UK Youth', said "There are 1.6 million children from a vulnerable family background for whom support is either patchy or non-existent. Just over half of these children are 'invisible' to services. Youth work could be the only answer to helping these children; a preventative service that provides support before problems arise."

'UK Youth' is a leading charity working across the UK. Their website states that "We have influence as a sector-supporting infrastructure body, a direct delivery partner and a campaigner for social change."

UK Youth's new 2025 strategy, "Unlocking Youth Work" outlines a bold ambition to impact young lives by unlocking youth work as a catalyst for change. "We will work in partnership to build a cross-sector movement, creating a society that understands, champions, and delivers effective youth work for all."

The more research I do for this book the more inspiring charities I discover which are doing such valuable work for our young people and which are needed now more than ever before.

The preliminary data, which was at the centre of a more in-depth report published later in 2021, is in line with recent research by the 'National Youth Agency' which found many youth charities are "running on empty".

"Youth services simply do not have the capacity or enough funding to meet young people's vastly increased needs," said the NYA's chief executive, Leigh Middleton. "They have depleted reserves and incomes slashed by half or more. We are calling for greater investment in frontline youth services right now, sustained throughout any lockdown and regional tier emergency measures."

Anne Longfield, the former Children's Commissioner for England, said the research was "shocking but sadly, not surprising".

****

As we look to the nation's recovery, Labour is clear that an ambitious plan for children must be at its heart. On the 8th June 2022 **Labour Children's Recovery Plan** was passed in Parliament.

They have an ambitious vision for every child, teenager and young adult growing up in the UK. This report builds on the vision Keir Starmer set out at 'Labour Connected', a speech he gave in 2020 where he set out plans to close the education gap so every child's future is determined by their potential, not their postcode.

The package of measures set out in this report give schools the resources to provide every child with new opportunities to socialise, learn and develop post-pandemic; working to reverse the gap in learning which has widened during the pandemic ensuring every child has the chance to reach their potential. With extracurricular activities, mental health support in schools and small group teaching available to all pupils who will benefit, Labour will prioritise children's wellbeing and social development as an essential part of supporting learning. As this report says, "Children and young people are excited to be back with their friends in school and feel ambitious and optimistic about their futures. Labour's plan matches this ambition, putting children at the heart of our national recovery."

They promise:-

- Breakfast clubs and new activities for every child: boost time for children to play and socialise after months away from their friends by enabling schools to offer an expanded range of extracurricular activities, from breakfast clubs to sport and drama, book clubs and debating societies;

- Quality mental health support in every school: give every child the support they need to transition back to school and manage personal challenges, with access to qualified in-school counselling staff alongside boosting wellbeing through extra activities;

- Make small group teaching available to all children who need it not just 1%, by reforming the Government's failing tutoring programme so no child falls behind because of pandemic disruption;

- Continued development for teachers: Teachers and school staff have had one of the toughest years of their careers - it is only by supporting them with training to stay on top of the latest knowledge and techniques that we can give every child a brilliant classroom experience;

- Invest in an Education Recovery Premium: support every child to reach their potential by investing in children who have faced the greatest disruption during the pandemic from early years to further education, and double the Pupil Premium for children in key transition years, delivering additional support for children who need it most;

- Ensure no child goes hungry during the pandemic by extending free school meals over the holidays, including the summer holidays.

This might indeed all be difficult to achieve straight away but at least it is a plan. All the Conservatives are offering is the failed catch-up tutoring programme.

Head teachers said they were "hugely disappointed" by a £1.4bn Covid recovery package, which was announced in June 2021 and which breaks down to £50 extra per pupil per year. The Education Policy Institute, which warned primary pupils had lost up to two months of learning in reading and three months in maths, said the extra funding was a tenth of what it estimated was needed.

Spread over three years, the extra cash is worth about 1% of the annual schools budget, they said.

****

They could also be doing much more about the horrific rise in knife crime by young people.

According to a report by the Office for National Statistics the number of people killed with a knife in England and Wales in 2021/22 was the highest on record for 76 years. Patrick Green, chief executive of anti-knife crime charity the 'Ben Kinsella Trust' cited the effects of the Covid-19 pandemic as a reason for knife crime rising faster amongst teenagers than any other age group. Mr Green told the *PA News Agency*: "As we emerged from Covid restrictions and those restrictions were lifted, we were seeing more evidence of young people made more vulnerable by Covid. Gangs are particularly good at picking up on vulnerabilities, are quick to pick them up and indeed lure young people and exploit them in criminal acts. We think there could be a link there."

Absolutely there could. This is another inspirational charity doing invaluable work for our young people.

They say that "We educate young people on the dangers of knife crime and help them to make positive choices to stay safe. Our workshops follow the journey of both the victim and the offender through a series of unique and immersive experiences to show young people how choices and consequences are intrinsically linked. Our workshops change young people's attitudes to knife crime; debunking the myth that carrying a knife will protect you. They strengthen peer values; ensuring young people give better advice to each other and challenge peers who are carrying (or thinking of carrying) a knife".

And former Children's Commissioner, Anne Longfield, said that "Areas suffering the most significant cuts in spending on young people have recorded larger increases in knife crime and drug-related crimes". She goes on to say "Youth services are the last line of defence for vulnerable children. If these children have a bad time at home and don't have the structure of school, for whatever reason, and then you take away youth services too, they're completely on their own, with nothing protecting them from physical abuse, self-harm and drug use, being exploited and groomed."

Matthew Hussey, the public affairs manager of the 'Children's Society,' said another missed opportunity was the Chancellor's spending review in December 2021.

"It was a chance to place children's services, which include council-led support for young people like youth work, on a sustainable footing and give councils the resources they need to rebuild the support so needed by children and young people," he said.

The 'Children's Society' says on their website that, "We are a national charity working to transform the hopes and happiness of young people facing abuse, exploitation and neglect. We support them through their most serious life challenges and we campaign tirelessly for the big social changes that will improve the lives of those who need hope most. We've been doing this for 140 years and we won't stop until we've built a society where hope is alive in every child."

So many of these wonderful charities are finding it so difficult after the pandemic when the government neglected the needs of children.

And here is the voice of a father who lost his son in a stabbing and who said that the closing down of youth centres across the country is "pushing children to violence".

Dwayne Roye, a community activist from Croydon, spoke to *Sky News* when he said he had "hosted his seventh annual football tournament today (22nd May 2022) to raise awareness about knife crime."

He manages Elite Development FC, a youth football team in Croydon, and he firmly believes budget cuts that have decimated youth services in parts of England - particularly south London - are linked to the rise in knife crime.

He told *Sky News*: "Every borough used to have a community centre - Brixton, Peckham, Croydon - but now they've all been shut down and this has had a terrible impact on our communities."

The government says there is extra money going into youth services but UNISON's head of local government Mike Short described the extra money from government as "a drop in the ocean".

"It won't cover the scale of damage caused by austerity," Mr Short told *Sky News*

"If ministers want to tackle crime, they need to rebuild youth services. And that means investing much more than they've promised."

That seems to be the on-going mantra that we hear all the time.

London is particularly hit hard as more than 40 per cent of London's youth clubs could close within a year because they have run out of money, research suggests.

A survey of more than 120 youth organisations by the charity 'London Youth' found that 43% said they will not be able to meet operational costs without securing additional funding for more than 12 months.

Of those, 14% said they face closure within three months. More than one quarter of clubs said they will have to make some staff redundant.

The figures highlight the devastating impact the pandemic has had on the sector.

'London Youth' said youth organisations were already facing severe budget cuts before the pandemic and their finances are now under even greater strain. It called for the Government to deliver the £500 million Youth Investment Fund, which they promised in the 2019 manifesto, to rescue the sector.

Rosemary Watt-Wyness, chief executive of 'London Youth' said: "This has been a very difficult year for young Londoners and the organisations that support them.

All young Londoners, no matter where they live, should be able to rely on high-quality youth services in their community."

'London Youth' supports the contribution of community-based youth clubs and youth workers, providing them with information, advice, and a wide range of accredited training. 'London Youth' works directly with young people to create "eye-catching and innovative" new opportunities in partnership with youth clubs at its outdoor activity and training centres. The group also advocates on behalf of its members.

So I think everyone agrees that the lack of support for youth services, particularly after the devastation of the pandemic together with increased mental health problems of children, are one of the main causes of increased violence amongst young people.

Oh no, wait a moment. I see a small paragraph in the *Times* today (9th October 2023) that the Chief Constable of Manchester Police told a fringe event at the Conservative Party Conference that actually **three year olds should be taught about criminal gangs to prevent them from being sucked into a life of crime** when they are older. So **that's** the problem then. He goes on to say, "We are growing a generation who have never had anyone saying 'no' to them."

Oh, of course, come on parents, and in particular you mothers out there, it's all your fault. Why did no-one think of that before?

Mr. Chief Constable, our children have had the word 'no' said to them every single day during the pandemic. Now, many of them are being told 'no, you can't have any food to eat, no you can't have a bed to sleep in, no there is no soap to wash with, nor shoes to put on your feet. Three year olds? What planet are you on Chief Constable?

****

But I see a really disturbing report today (12th November 2023). Mark Townsend writes in the *Observer* about a report by the 'Youth Endowment Fund'. This is the largest ever survey by government advisers to try to find out what drives knife crime, bullying and gang rivalries.

Perhaps the most upsetting and shocking finding is the fact that 358,000 teenagers had been physically injured during the last 12 months and one in five teenagers admitted to skipping school during the last 12 months because they felt unsafe.

The report criticises the government's approach to this problem which doesn't surprise me in the least.

They say they rely too heavily on granting police more powers instead of tackling the root causes. How many times do we hear that? It would appear that nine out of ten teenagers who committed violence that led to physical injury received no follow- up support whatsoever. Studies showed that indeed mentoring programmes can prevent violence to a significant degree. **So then comes the most damning sentence in the entire report. "On a positive note it does show that we could make a colossal difference if we wanted to."**

WHAT? Here you have an answer to some of the problems of knife crime and you are not bothered one way or the other? You sit there and say well we could sort this out I suppose but we will just throw some money at it and see what happens.

Well what happens is that fatal stabbings by children as young as 12 continue unabated due to the complete absence of concern and the gross incompetence of this government.

****

Then we continue to hear that more and more **school sports fields are being sold off**.

Altogether the government has approved the sale of 215 school playing fields in England since 2010 at a time when childhood obesity is reaching epidemic proportions, according to new research by the GMB union.

Toby Helm, political editor of the *Guardian*, writes on August 20th 2023 that the number of hours young people spend doing PE and sport in secondary schools in England has fallen by more than 12% since the 2012 London Olympics.

He recalls a speech given by David Cameron in 2012, when he was Prime Minister, when he said it was vital that the London Games spurred his government to improve the provision of sport in state schools, which he admitted had been underfunded for far too long. Cameron insisted there was "one area in particular where the Olympic spirit of taking part can make a real difference to young people. And that is school sport and helping to drive participation in sport itself."

His words were greeted with scepticism at the time by sports organisations, not least because his education secretary, **Michael Gove, had systematically dismantled a network of school sports partnerships set up by the Labour government, in order to save money, as one of his first acts at the Department for Education.**

So the mantra 'all words and no action' goes back to well before the pandemic.

******

Then there is the closure of public swimming pools. In the summer of 2022 the BBC found that between 2019 and 2022, one in six local authorities had seen at least one pool close, on either a permanent or temporary basis.

'Swim England' estimates that around 1 in 4 children currently leave primary school unable to swim 25m. That is a dreadful legacy to own. And that number is expected to rise to as many as 6 in 10 by 2025.

'Swim England' said more than five million swimming sessions were lost during the pandemic. Pools first had to close in March 2020.

Normally, 1.2 million children learn to swim each year through 'Swim England's' 'Learn To Swim' programme, but these opportunities have been significantly reduced as a result of the lockdowns and pool closures.

The importance of learning to swim is highlighted by the fact that drowning is the third highest cause of death in children in the UK. Drowning is not simply a case of avoiding swimming, as 40% of drowning victims never intended being in the water. Accidents leading to unexpected submersion (ie walkers, runners or other activities near water) mean that being able to swim is an essential lifesaving skill that should be integrated into every child's education.

These startling figures have been published by the 'All-Party Parliamentary Group for Swimming' as well as 'Swim England', who are warning of a 'lost generation' of swimmers unless action is taken to halt the projected decline.

In addition to this, we know from 'Swim England's Value of Swimming' report that swimmers have higher wellbeing than non-swimmers and are happier, and healthier. They also show higher levels of self-confidence and self-efficacy. The report also shows the benefits are particularly pronounced for girls – girls who swim have considerably higher increases in wellbeing, health and self-confidence compared to boys.

Teaching children to swim is one of the key drowning prevention interventions stated by The World Health Organisation (WHO, 2020), and a requirement of the UK Government. Failing to provide access to swimming pools and swimming lessons should be viewed as mass child neglect.

It is a tragedy that up to one million children have missed out on swimming lessons over the past year due to lockdowns (Swim England). Given the low base from which the UK entered the COVID-19 pandemic (one in three children unable to swim), they say that "we can ill-afford to allow the continued closure and permanent loss of access to swimming pools. In addition to the accepted benefits of physical activity for physical, mental, emotional and social health, swimming saves lives."

They say that, "almost 2,000 swimming pools in England could be closed by 2030 without urgent government action."

The number of quality facilities could drop by 40%, limiting access for competitive and recreational swimmers. It adds that pools built in the 1960s and 70s have not been refurbished at a sufficient rate and without investment of £1bn, it says there will be a "huge decline" in the availability of pools.

But in February of this year we get a stark warning from Community Leisure UK the industry body representing the operators of 880 pools across England, Scotland and Wales. They say that roughly half of the UK's community swimming pools face closure or service cuts within six months – placing thousands of jobs at risk – unless the Government steps in with urgent financial support to tackle crippling energy bills.

So what do we hear? We hear that the Government has revealed that following the conclusion of the current scheme, there will be a new 'Energy Bills Discount Scheme' which will come into effect from April 2023 and run for 12 months. This universal scheme is much less generous than previous support provided and **swimming pools and leisure centres have been excluded from extra support.**

Responding to the news, 'Swim England's chief executive Jane Nickerson, said: "This decision by the Government to not provide additional support to swimming pools and leisure centres is a hammer blow and flies in the face of previous statements from the Government about the importance of physical activity and reducing pressures on the NHS. The Government must urgently rethink and match their rhetoric around the importance of physical activity with action to provide the support that is so desperately needed to keep these vital facilities open for people to use. Failing to do so is just storing up much greater costs for the health and social care system."

Will Rishi Sunak listen and act? Hmmm. Not sure. He and his children are actually OK because at his mansion in leafy Richmond, Yorkshire, they have a new private swimming pool. Oh but that's not all. Apparently it uses so much energy that the local electricity network had to be upgraded to meet its power demands. Engineers had to install a substantial amount of equipment and a new connection to the National Grid that runs across open fields. This new pool was built on green-field agricultural land that until recently was used for grazing animals.

And only last month, the operators of a public swimming pool near the prime minister's home said it would reduce public access because of the increased cost of energy.

OK Rishi, maybe you could just listen to the voices of our children as they talk about what swimming means to them.

"The water is where I find my peace and strength. It's my happy place."

"In the water, you're weightless, free, and capable of anything."

"I love swimming because it's really fun and I get to play with my friends."

"Swimming is like flying in the water."

"I feel like a mermaid when I swim."

"Swimming is my favourite sport because it's a great way to cool off on a hot day."

Is anyone listening? Well maybe not about swimming pools but there is this:- In March of this year (2023) the Government's Youth Investment Fund have finally announced that young people are to benefit from the rebuilding and renovation of youth centres in some of the country's most disadvantaged areas, as they become beneficiaries of the first major tranche from this Fund .

"Every young person will have access to regular clubs and activities by 2025," a government spokesperson told *Sky News*, amid criticism about the number of centres which have closed over the past decade

Wow that is amazing and hopefully we can believe this. Well if it is left to local mayors I think we can. For I see this:

TOWER HAMLETS

On October 1st the borough's mayor of Tower Hamlets, Mr. Lutfur Rahman thinks that even with its surging population and rife child poverty, its £13.7m funding package will pay off. He says that the borough's population has swollen by 22% since 2011; its average age is 30, the youngest in the country; it has a child poverty rate of 56%, the highest in London; and 40,000 to 50,000 people there are thought to live in overcrowded homes. Investing in youth services is crucial – especially in Tower Hamlets.

"The kids don't have a proper space of their own," he said. "The link between schools, education, youth services and crime is so important. Give them good after-school provision, linked with schools, and they are bound to do well."

The move is intended to correct the decade of swingeing cuts to youth services. A 2022 YMCA report found that funding cuts in England had reached £1.1bn, representing a real-terms fall of 74%, since 2010-11.

The new events programme emphasises the post-16 transition into education, training and employment, alongside preventing young people from offending and entering the criminal justice system. The borough is hoping to position itself as a leader in child and youth services. The investment forms part of a wider package of public health initiatives, which includes £5.7m for universal free school meals for primary and secondary school pupils, £1.1m to re-introduce education maintenance allowances and university bursaries, and £730,000 for children with special educational and additional needs.

Ideally, Mr. Rahman wants to see more central government support for youth services, especially given the cost of living crisis.

Well yes don't we all? But this is a really good start and I can end this chapter on a more hopeful note as we watch to see what progress is made around the country to help all of our children to start to recover from the mistakes made during the pandemic.

****

*"If we could have but one generation
of properly born, trained, educated
and healthy children, a thousand other
problems of government would vanish."*

Herbert Hoover

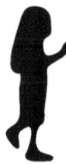

CHILDREN AND EDUCATION

THE CONSERVATIVE RECOVERY PROGRAMME

On **February 4th 2021** the most wonderful thing happened. Sir Kevan Collins was appointed as the government's school catch-up tsar following the Covid 19 nightmare. He proposed some great ideas which were music to my ears. He said that the school day should be extended by a couple of hours for things like music, sport, drama and general health and well-being. Teachers need not be involved but volunteers and club leaders could be brought in.

On **June 3rd, just four months later, he resigned**. I heard this on the news at 5.30pm and I was shocked. He had asked the Treasury for £15 billion over three years and was offered £1.4 billion. What an insult. An insult not just to Sir Kevan but to all the children and teachers in our state schools.

He stated in his resignation letter that "the average primary school will receive just £50 per child per year."

"Above all" he states **"I am concerned that the package that was announced betrays an undervaluation of the importance of education."**

And everything that follows in this chapter re-enforces the truth of this statement.

So who was the Chancellor at that time who decided that our children and our schools did not need sufficient funds to enable a first-class education? Oh yes of course........Rishi Sunak ....whose daughters, by the way, attend a private school.

Anne Longfield, former Children's Commissioner, refers to this when reporting to the Covid inquiry in 2022.

"Kevan Collins' multi- billion-pound recovery programme was drawn up at the request of the Prime Minister and would have had a really significant impact on children's lives, not only to recover from the pandemic, but also to help them bounce back to a better place," she said. "But it was turned down and replaced with a very narrow, much cheaper option. That was another huge mistake."

But that is how much this government thinks our children are worth.

****

Schools continue to be under-funded and under-resourced which has resulted in many strikes from desperate staff. Head teachers are breaking down in tears, suffering migraines and even passing out, with six in 10 admitting they have considered changing jobs in the past year because of increased level of stress.

The head of a state school in Cumbria shared the resignation letter she sent recently to her board of governors with the *Observer*. "The last two and a half years have been the toughest I have ever known," the letter begins. "The experience has almost broken me, and the situation shows no signs of improving."

She wrote that she is "exhausted by the continued battles" as a result of 10 years of cuts to school funding and the "relentless reduction" of other public services supposed to be helping children and their families.

Her letter ends: "I no longer want to work for a government that is so out of touch with reality and treats my profession and our children with such contempt."

Brian Walton, head teacher at Brookside Academy in Street, Somerset, says running a school should be "the best job in the world", but he plans to resign this year because he thinks "the whole system is broken". "I've been a head teacher for 20 years and I've never seen anything like this," he says.

He also says that he has never seen so many of their families relying on food banks. "People are coping with anxiety and mental health problems. Behaviour problems in school are really escalating."

Sinéad McBrearty, chief executive of 'Education Support', the charity which supports school leaders with their mental health, says: "Heads are at risk of heart attacks and strokes. They are asking 'Do I choose my career or my health?'."

I look up 'Education Support' and find their web site which says that:-

"We support individuals and help schools, colleges and universities to improve the mental health and wellbeing of their staff. We also carry out research and advocate for changes in Government policy for the benefit of the education workforce."

Well as a retired primary school teacher I never knew there was a charity like this. But then I am talking about a long time ago when teachers were respected and schools were properly funded.

And of course children are still going to school hungry. More and more, teachers are having to use their own money to buy children food and also sometimes shoes. They are having to be social workers as well as teachers.

An estimated 800,000 children in poverty do not qualify for free school meals. To be eligible households must have an annual income of under £7,400 before benefits and after tax. That threshold has been frozen since 2018, even though prices have risen since then.

The number of UK children in food poverty has nearly doubled in the last year to almost 4 million, new data shows, ramping up pressure on ministers to expand the provision of free school meals to struggling families.

Aha wait a moment. I hear the Tory MP for Bury, James Daly, say that the children who are struggling in his constituency are doing so due to "crap parenting." Hmm. The Tory mantra appears to be always blame others and whilst I dislike writing language such as this I think it is important that we all know the extent of the insults and ignorance of those who put themselves forward to represent us in positions of power.

****

On top of all this we are hearing that the Government has scrapped a £5m plan to fund a "school cooking revolution".

In February 2022, the Government announced plans for a school cooking revolution as part of its levelling up agenda. The scheme aimed to tackle the country's rising child obesity problem. This was a wonderful idea and was greeted with positivity and acclaim.

So what happens? Just 19 months later it is abandoned. Why? The Department for Education said that it would not be taking this forward because it was "in favour of using an existing, established route for developing curriculum content, while not diverting resource from wider curriculum commitments outlined in the Schools White Paper." In other words they are not prepared to spend further money on our children.

School charities have said they are disappointed by the U-turn. Naomi Duncan, the head of 'Chefs in Schools', said: "We're extremely disheartened to hear of the abandonment of yet another pledge relating to child health. Without investing in the training of school leaders and teaching staff, empowering them to drive forward food education, we'll further fail the next generation – who are already on the front line of the food-related disease crisis."

The head of 'School Food Matters', Stephanie Slater, said she believes the Government has done little to invest in cooking and food education.

Ms. Slater said: "Delivery of food education has been patchy so the £5m promised in the levelling up white paper was a welcome boost and suggested that the Department for Education was at last understanding the value of food education. Sadly it seems that once more, charities are being left to plug gaps in education and to provide opportunities for school children to learn the life skills they need for their long-term health and happiness."

As I keep finding out, this country relies heavily on charities to do the work which should be done by the government.

It would appear that there is never any money for our schools.

****

DANGEROUS INFRASTRUCTURE

But for goodness-sake what on earth is this? On Thursday 31st August 2023 schools which were due to start the new school year the following Monday were told they would have to begin the autumn term taking lessons remotely or in temporary buildings after **the government ordered more than 100 schools to immediately shut buildings made with aerated concrete RAAC, that is liable to sudden collapse.**

This is unbelievable. This has been known about for years but this government has chosen to do absolutely nothing until literally the last minute.

These schools are at risk of causing fatal injury with collapsing ceilings and the exposure of asbestos.

Geoff Wilkinson, a senior building inspector, said: "The risk has been known about for decades. There should have been an ongoing maintenance plan for these buildings to be upgraded and replaced over the last 40 years. They are all past their serviceable lifetime. It's shocking to discover that the maintenance plan wasn't in place and there hadn't been a programme of demolitions."

At least 13 schools affected by the failing concrete crisis were included in the school rebuilding programme scrapped by Michael Gove in 2010. Labour had a £55bn 'Building Schools for the Future' programme, according to the BBC but it was this that was scrapped by Gove as soon as the Tories came to power.

In fact more than 700 rebuilding or refurbishment projects were shelved by the Conservative-led coalition government as part of efforts to bring down net borrowing, which had peaked in 2010 at £152bn.

Gove, who was education secretary at the time, had described this building programme as plagued by "massive overspends, tragic delays, botched construction projects and needless bureaucracy". But Geoff Barton, general secretary of the Association of School and College Leaders, told BBC that while the programme was expensive and over ambitious "it was saying something important that the nation's schools needed to be refurbished. What we've got today in some of those schools is head teachers scrambling around trying to identify concrete that might look like Aero bars when they should be focusing on children's learning and development."

He called the crisis over RAAC a "national scandal", adding that the 13 schools would not be facing disruption if the coalition government had not cancelled the BSF programme.

The roof of a primary school in Kent actually collapsed for goodness sake, in 2018, when there were repeated warnings and calls for action, but nothing was done. The mantra of the Conservative party.

Ministers have been accused of gross incompetence and the Prime Minister was forced to deny claims by a former top civil servant that he had ignored warnings over a "critical risk to life" by cutting school repairs funding when he was still Chancellor.

"Children will always be our top priority" they keep saying. Lies and more lies.

But of course we have to hear from the present Education Secretary. This is what she should have said:-

"I am extremely sorry that we have failed our children in such a dangerous way. Our incompetence and neglect has been unprecedented and I do agree that we should all resign forthwith."

But no of course she didn't say that. Her name is Gillian Keegan and in an extraordinary outburst which left No 10 reeling, she actually said others had "sat on their a***" over the crisis and she had done a "f****** good job".

Where do these people come from?

Former Department for Education mandarin Jonathan Slater claimed that when he was Chancellor, Mr Sunak had blocked a bid to get ahead of the crisis by rebuilding up to 400 schools each year. Accusing the Tories of putting a pledge to build new "free schools" over the safety of children, Mr Slater said the rebuilding programme was cut to just 50 schools per year. Mr Sunak scrambled to distance himself from the claim, saying Mr Slater was "completely and utterly wrong".

However it emerged just four schools in the main rebuild programme have been completed in the past two years, adding to the pressure on Rishi Sunak. Then we hear Ms. Keegan ordering school leaders to get "off their backsides" to help sort out the chaos.

Yes, well that has gone down well with our teachers.

****

DIRTY, HUNGRY AND TIRED

We have all heard of food poverty but there is now something else which schools have to cope with which is **hygiene poverty.**

Julie McCulloch, the director of policy at the Association of School and College Leaders, said: "Hygiene poverty is linked to very high levels of deprivation as families struggle with the cost of things like washing machines, energy bills and clothes. Many schools routinely help out by discreetly washing clothes and providing items of uniform."

There is now a hygiene bank where people can donate new and unused goods such as deodorants, shower gel, soap, shampoo, and laundry detergent.

There is a stigma to not being able to keep clean and so it is not discussed very much but it can have a huge impact on the self-esteem and mental health of a child

Many children are bullied because of it and many will not invite friends to their house because they are ashamed.

And then I hear about this. A dishwasher tablet manufacturer, SMOL, has created a scheme called 'Suds in Schools Project'. They are creating **free-to-use school laundrettes,** to enable children living in hygiene poverty to access clean clothes with their help. They say that "All donations received are put straight into helping kit out and install new washer-dryers into schools in suitable locations across the UK. Then for the length that the scheme is required SMOL will provide the detergent to schools for free."

I am actually in shock hearing about this but I have to congratulate SMOL for this scheme.

****

Oh no! I now hear of another phrase which is "**bed poverty**". This is our children we are talking about here.

'Banardo's' state that more than a million children in the UK either sleep on the floor or share a bed with parents or siblings because their family cannot afford the "luxury" of replacing broken frames and mouldy linen.

The charity says increasing "bed poverty" reflects growing levels of destitution in which low-income families already struggling with soaring food or gas bills often find they are also unable to afford a comfortable night's sleep.

So some of our children are arriving at school hungry, dirty and exhausted.

****

But then some of our children are not arriving in school at all.

ABSENTEEISM

More than 140,000 schoolchildren in England were officially "severely absent" in the summer term of 2022, according to official Department of Education figures - and the number of these pupils, missing at least 50% of classes, is growing.

They are away from school for a variety of reasons - including anxiety and mental health, special educational needs and disabilities.

Many of them stopped attending school during the pandemic - never to return. And now, they are not really on anyone's radar.

Anne Longfield now chairs the 'Commission on Young Lives' - an independent commission that looks to prevent crises in vulnerable young people.

She is concerned that the number of children not attending school will put young people at risk of serious violence and exploitation. She warns there is an "avalanche of inequalities" worsened by the cost-of-living crisis and the pandemic that is putting children at higher risk.

While not all children who are persistently absent are being exploited, Ms. Longfield warns that missing school heightens the risk.

Of course it does and there is not sufficient data at the moment to identify these children. An enormous amount of work needs to be done in order to find them and support them and their families. There needs to be a concerted approach by social workers, mentors, district nurses, GPs, mental health workers and local authorities to try to locate these families and children in order to support them and help them in every way they need.

But "ooh yes, this is dreadful and their parents need to be fined," coo our millionaire MPs. Their stupidity is indeed 'world beating'. These families need practical solutions, financial input, care and kindness.

****

But then I see this.

HOME SCHOOL REGISTER

In **April 2019** Damian Hinds, the then education secretary, (there have been 13 since 2010) announced that parents would be required to register home-educated children with their local authority under government proposals intended to prevent young people from disappearing off the radar.

I am dumbfounded. Apparently no-one has any true idea how many children are absent from school because **there is no available data on the number of children, who are being home-schooled.**

Damian Hinds said: "As a government, we have a duty to protect our young people and do our utmost to make sure they are prepared for life in modern Britain.

"That's why this register of children not in school is so important: not to crack down on those dedicated parents doing an admirable job of educating their children in their own homes, but to prevent vulnerable young people from vanishing under the radar."

"Under the proposals, which will be subject to a 12-week consultation, it will be parents' responsibility to register their child if they are not being taught in a state-funded or registered independent school."

So I make 12 weeks from April 2019 about September 2019.

Well The Local Government Association, which represents councils, welcomed the register, but called on the government to go further and give local authorities the powers and funding to enter homes or other premises to check a child's schooling. Without those powers – and more funding to enact them – the LGA says concerns will persist for a minority of children who could be at risk of neglect or poor future prospects.

The children's charity 'NSPCC' said a register alone would not automatically safeguard children. "There must also be regular checks just like any other education setting to ensure that children are being properly looked after when they learn," a spokesperson said.

Head of Ofsted and chief inspector of schools in England, Amanda Spielman, said: "Ofsted has long had concerns about the increasing numbers of school-age children not attending a registered school, many of whom may not be receiving a high-quality education or being kept safe.

"We are especially concerned about children 'off-rolled' from schools, and those in illegal schools. The new register will make it easier to detect and tackle these serious problems."

So there we are. Much talk and discussion and so let us look for this register. It must have been especially useful during the pandemic.

As I dig and delve to try to find out more information about it I see this headline in the *Guardian* written on **February 3rd 2022** by Sally Weale, their education correspondent.

"Government is planning compulsory national register but details of penalties are yet to be determined."

What? But they were talking about this three years before in 2019.

Ms. Weale goes on to say "**Ministers have promised to bring forward legislation at the earliest opportunity,** but the government's response on Thursday to a 2019 public consultation on the issue said the rollout was still "subject to securing the necessary resources", and details of what penalties parents may face have yet to be determined."

Oh for goodness sake that is ridiculous.

And then this just gets worse and worse.

In **May this year (2023**) we heard that Conservative MP Flick Drummond tabled a new Bill aimed at placing a legal duty on local authorities to maintain a register of children who are not in school. She said that child safety concerns sparked calls in Parliament for a register of home-schooled children to be established. Apparently she said "there could be up to 81,000 children in England who are being home schooled, but "no one knows how they are being educated".

She went on to say "Now, many of those, of course, will be well-educated because their parents are doing a brilliant job. But there are an awful lot of children that aren't. And the local authorities at the moment have no right to actually go in and see how they are being educated, which is extraordinary."

No Ms. Drummond, what is extraordinary is that this register still doesn't exist after four years of empty promises, dither and delay.

And here it is again on **November 9th 2023** as we listen to the debate on the King's Speech when the Education Secretary (now Gillian Keegan) has reaffirmed the Government's pledge to establish a register for children not in school, but without specifying a time frame for legislation.

Can you believe it? Still no firm commitment. Somewhere I wrote the words "at the earliest opportunity" but obviously that has no meaning at all to Conservatives.

There is much criticism of course as Ms. Drummond expressed her disappointment. She said that "Parents have a right to homeschool children, and my Bill would have done nothing to prevent them. Its aim is to ensure that vulnerable children are identifiable and can be supported. There is a crisis in attendance post-Covid and we have to tackle it before these children miss out. My Bill fell at the end of the last session and I noted that the schools minister committed to introduce legislation at a future suitable opportunity. What more suitable opportunity could there be than the one that we have now? So I was deeply disappointed at the lack of the Bill in the gracious speech."

Also Lib Dem education spokeswoman Munira Wilson asked for an explanation as to why the previously promised register had not been addressed in the Government's plans for the parliamentary year.

Well explanation there was none and many children continue to be lost in the wilderness under a government that shows no care, nor concern, nor interest in them whatsoever.

****

And then I see this.

GOVERNMENT CENSORSHIP

An *Observer* investigation has discovered that experts who criticised state education policy online had their posts monitored by the Department for Education who then tried to cancel a conference where some of these "unsuitable" speakers were due to take part.

Ruth Swailes and Aaron Bradbury, co-authors of a bestselling book on early childhood, were told by the organisers of a government-sponsored event for childminders and nursery workers, which they were due to speak at in March, that the DfE planned to cancel the conference just days before it opened because they were deemed to be "unsuitable" headline speakers.

What on earth is going on here?

Speaking to the *Observer*, Dr. Bradbury, principal lecturer in early childhood studies at Nottingham Trent University, said: "I received a phone call from the organisers saying there were some concerns about us being speakers. The DfE had decided we were unsuitable because we had been critical of government policy."

He said: "To be told that we couldn't have this debate felt like we were living in a dictatorship, not a democracy. **We were due to talk about nurturing and early child development. It wasn't some covert stuff about infiltrating Russia.**"

Ms.Swailes, an independent consultant who advises schools and nurseries on early years' education, was so shocked that she filed a subject access request, requiring the DfE to disclose any documents it held on her.

The results, which she received at the end of the summer (2023) revealed that the department kept a file on her. It included critical tweets she had posted about Ofsted, and noted that she had "liked" posts promoting guidance on teaching young children that was written by educationists rather than the government.

She said: "They have tried to silence me. What they did could have ruined my livelihood and still has the potential to."

The event was eventually allowed to go ahead after Ms. Swailes and Ms. Bradbury threatened the department with legal action, although, listen to this, a senior government official was present to "monitor" what they said.

If you are not disgusted and extremely concerned about this then I think you might need to read that again.

Dr. Ian Cushing, a senior lecturer in critical applied linguistics, at Manchester Metropolitan University revealed that both the DfE and Ofsted were monitoring him and, said: "What is deeply troubling to me is the fact that they spend substantial amounts of time and money in these surveillance procedures at a time when schools are being hit by economic difficulties and cost of living crises."

Sue Cowley, an education expert who runs training for schools, tweeted her response to the records she had been sent under her name this week: "Excuse my language but WTAF [what the actual fuck] are the DfE doing spending taxpayer money conducting surveillance on critics of government policy on here?"

When asked why the government had been compiling files on the social media activity of its critics, the DfE said it did not comment on individual cases.

Big Brother is alive and well in 21st century Conservative Britain.

******

LITERACY

I was shocked to hear that one in seven primary schools have no library provision. Some will have a few books in the classrooms but many of the books will be in a poor condition. I then see a report by the Primary School Library Alliance which is supported by the National Literacy Trust.

The 'National Literacy Trust' is an independent charity that empowers children, young people, and adults, with the literacy skills they need to succeed. They do an enormous amount of work in schools especially in order to help young people to read. They say that "one in seven primary schools in England do not have a library and over three-quarters of a million children in the UK do not have access to books that we know enable better educational outcomes and greater well-being. There is no statutory requirement for schools to have a library."

Through their 'Primary Schools Alliance' they want to help transform 1,000 primary school libraries by 2025, giving them the books, training and support they need.

They commissioned the largest UK survey on the issue of school libraries in partnership with the 'Great School Libraries Campaign'. Overall, 3,752 or almost 1 in 5 state primary schools across England, Scotland, Northern Ireland and Wales answered a range of school library related questions between July 2022 and September 2022.

On their website the 'Great School Libraries Campaign' say that "Great School Libraries is a three year evidence-based campaign to bring back libraries and access to librarians in every school in the UK. Our guiding principle is a firm belief that every child deserves a great school library. Phase 1 of the campaign launched in September 2018 will run until the summer of 2021. Phase 2 of the Campaign launched in the spring of 2022 will run until the summer of 2025."

So yet another inspirational charity trying to alleviate the government's shortcomings

This survey showed that only 86% of state primary schools across the UK said they have a designated school library area.

These are the percentages of regions in England that do **not** have a designated library area.

North East 18%
North West 16%
West Midlands 13%
East Midlands 12%
Yorkshire & the Humber 12%
South West 9%
London 8%
East of England 7%
South East 6%

And this is heart- breaking to read. The head of English in a primary school said:- "For children who live and go to school in typically disadvantaged areas, it's a very real possibility that they may go through their entire childhood and not own a single book...Having access to a school library can be absolutely vital in their development and well-being."

The challenge of transforming and sustaining primary school libraries is a large-scale challenge and this report clearly sets out the gap in provision.

This is even more challenging for the 1 in 11 children and young people from disadvantaged backgrounds who say they don't have a book of their own at home , where school is often the first opportunity for children to discover the magic and benefits of reading.

Here are the voices from some children talking about how important a designated reading space is to them.

"I like going to the school reading space because it's a calm, relaxing space where you can chill out, read and let the book come to life."

"I love our school library because it's got so many sections and choices of lots of amazing books."

"My favourite book is an emotional book...It takes me to another world."

By mid-2023 the Trust had helped 500 schools.

By mid-2025 they hope to have helped 1,000 schools.

The report concludes with the following words:-

"In the Schools White Paper, the government set a target of 90% of primary school children reaching the expected standard in reading by 2030. The government can signal its commitment to this target by supporting the development of primary school libraries in the following ways:

1.   The Secretary of State for Education publicly acknowledging the positive role that primary school libraries can play in boosting literacy and endorse the aims and approach of the 'Primary School Library Alliance.'

2.   The Department for Education committing to ensuring that every primary school has a library by 2025 and publish an action plan setting out how it will work in partnership with others to achieve this goal.

3.   The Department for Education working with the' Primary School Library Alliance' to agree upon a sustainable, long-term funding model. For example, the introduction of a government matched funding programme, in which the government pays a proportion of the total costs, could help to leverage further private sector investment and secure high-quality resources.

By working together, we can ensure that every child, no matter their background, has access to books that are engaging and inspiring. We hope the government will support us in this endeavour. We would welcome a positive dialogue with the Department for Education."

But this government does not like talking to anyone.

I find it unbelievable that this prime minister can talk about introducing compulsory maths until 18, a baccalaureate instead of A levels, and better skill based education when schools are in complete melt- down and they don't have enough books.

****

And they don't have enough teachers.

EXHAUSTED TEACHERS

The retention and recruitment of teachers is an ongoing problem. In the primary sector, 59% of senior leaders indicate a decrease in the number of applicants compared to the usual, slightly higher than the 54%, reported last year. In the secondary sector, the recruitment cycle appears to be even more challenging, with over 80% of leaders stating a decrease in applicants compared to the norm, a notable increase from 65% reporting the same last year.

But just today (4th October 2023) we hear a speech by Rishi Sunak at the Conservative Party Conference where he says that education is the most important thing to him and he wants to make our education system the best in the world. Well if he acknowledges all the above, most of which has happened under his watch, he has his work cut out.

But he has just announced that certain specialist teachers will get a bonus of £30,000 for their first five years in the job. That is £500 a month. Well that should do it. And anything for other teachers Mr. Sunak? Just asking for a nation. How about paying them all a decent salary?

And I see a report by the Institute for Fiscal Studies which has just said that costs faced by schools are growing faster than inflation making their budgets worth less than in 2010. It says that **"the purchasing power of school spending per pupil in 2024-2025 will be about 3 percent lower than in 2009-2010"**

But just in case you have forgotten, this is what Ministers think of you teachers out there. Gavin Williamson, when Education Secretary during the pandemic, made the decision to delay A levels exams for a few weeks due to the virus. **So Matt Hancock the health secretary wrote to him and said: "Cracking announcement today. What a bunch of absolute arses the teaching unions are."**

To which Sir Gavin responded: "I know they really, really do just hate work."

Mr. Hancock's reply was two laughing face emojis and a bullseye.

Teaching morale is at an all-time low with teachers burnt out and stressed and children are faced with being taught in tents and porta cabins because their schools are falling down.

This is the reality facing our schools at the moment. Read and despair.

****

FUNDING RESOURCES

And then despair some more. There is a headline in the *Guardian* today (6th October 2023) which reads:

England's schools to be given less money after DfE admits bungling figures."

"Bungling" is a very appropriate adjective. It sums up the Department for Education perfectly.

There appears to have been a mistake made due to an underestimate of pupil numbers meaning that the amount schools receive for each pupil will be lower than previously announced. So head teachers who have already worked out how to spend their budgets for 2024-2025 will now have to redraw it as they will be given at least £50 less for each pupil.

For a typical secondary school the loss equates to a teacher's salary.

"Chaos at the heart of government" is the response from Paul Whiteman general secretary of the National Association of Head Teachers.

The Institute of Fiscal Studies had already warned that the purchasing powers of school spending a pupil in 2024 -2025 would be about 3% lower than in 2009-10 because of rising costs.

The anger from schools is palpable.

****

AT WAR WITH THE UNIONS
19TH OCTOBER 2023

Collapse-prone concrete has been found in 43 more schools in England, bringing the total number affected to 217.

Some have still not returned to normal teaching - with education unions calling out the government for not offering a clear timeline for when repair work will be completed.

And as we approach half term our Education secretary Gillian Keegan says:

"Well done all you teachers and teaching assistants for all your incredible hard work educating and nurturing our young children. As you approach half term I know you all deserve a much needed rest because it is so difficult to work in a system that has been starved of resources and money. Children are being taught specialist subjects by non-specialist teachers and the children are hungry and have anxiety issues. You all deserve a medal or at least a decent pay rise."

Oh no. Wait a minute. That was the script which she must have mis-laid. That was what she **should** have said. What she **actually** said was "if you go on strike you will get the sack," or words to that effect.

The crass ignorance and incompetence of our education secretary is beyond belief.

She actually announced that she would be discussing with the Unions plans that could be put in place to assure minimum staffing levels during any future strikes. This will be on a voluntary basis at first but in future she could, if they don't comply, use the powers given to her by the Minimum Service Levels Act passed earlier this year to force them.

Yes well that hasn't gone down well. It is mainly because there are **not** minimum staffing levels that they have **gone** on strike.

The unions are spitting mad and Daniel Kebede, general secretary of the National Education Union says that the government has no mandate whatsoever "to implement such an attack on our democratic freedoms".

Geoff Barton, general secretary of the Association of School and College Leaders said that the government should be supporting the profession. "By attempting to remove the right to strike instead of engaging with the profession and seeking to address their concerns, the secretary of state demonstrates that her priorities are in completely the wrong place," he said.

The National Association of Head Teachers union said it was an "overtly hostile act from the government and an attack on the basic democratic freedoms of school leaders and teachers".

Many teachers are saying that we need an ex-teacher or ex-head teacher as our education secretary. Well at the very least maybe just someone who knows about teaching.

And I say what on earth does she think she is doing? Is she really saying that she will use force if necessary? Will she really sack teachers? Well she will have to move fast because they are all leaving in droves and very soon there will be no teachers left to sack.

So our education system is still in crisis, our children are suffering and this government appears to be unconcerned.

****

ONLINE PROTECTION

But I **will** write about good news when I see it. At last, today, (24th October 2023) the **Online Safety Act has become law in the UK, after years of dither and delay. This Act introduces new rules which require social media companies to remove illegal content and protect children from 'harmful' material.**

There has been so much debate about freedom of speech etc and so much prevarication due to the rapid turnover of ministers that this bill should have been passed years ago.

Apparently 'WhatsApp' had threatened to withdraw from the UK rather than abide by these rules.

So according to the GOV.UK website this Bill is designed to:

Make social media companies legally responsible for keeping children and young people safe online.

It will protect children by making social media platforms:

- *remove illegal content quickly or prevent it from appearing in the first place. This includes removing content promoting self-harm*

- *prevent children from accessing harmful and age-inappropriate content*

- *enforce age limits and age-checking measures*

- *ensure the risks and dangers posed to children on the largest social media platforms are more transparent, including by publishing risk assessments*

- *provide parents and children with clear and accessible ways to report problems online when they do arise*

OK 'WhatsApp', which bit of these aims do you disagree with?

The 'NSPCC' have welcomed this result and say that it "will mean that children up and down the UK are fundamentally safer in their everyday lives." Their chief executive, Peter Wanless, said in a statement. "Tech companies will be legally compelled to protect children from sexual abuse and avoidable harm."

'Barnardo's' chief executive Lynn Perry said: "The Online Safety Act is an important first step towards making the UK the safest place for a child to be online."

Well yes it is a first step as it is to be implemented in three stages because nothing is ever done as a matter of urgency by this government but I repeat: it is a start.

Those that fail to comply will face fines of up to £18 million or 10% of annual global revenue, meaning potentially billions of pounds for the biggest firms.

In the most extreme cases, tech bosses could even face prison.

****

TERTIARY EDUCATION

Then we listen to the voices of our university students.

Costs of renting student accommodation has risen by nearly £1,000 over the last year. Many students are left with about 50p a week from the maintenance loan in order to pay their rent. So many are very depressed at not being able to find anywhere to live and many are travelling miles because they are forced to continue living with their parents. They can't socialise or join sports teams and they spend much of their time trying to find suitable accommodation.

"This has put so much stress on my mental health as I'm spending all my time looking for accommodation – which is either too expensive or too far away," says one first year student. *"I've given up on the expected first year experience."*

The **National Student Accommodation Survey 2023** by Laura Brown in 'Student Accommodation, Student Money Surveys' which was updated on the 8th February 2023, talks to many students and finds a worrying trend about accommodation difficulties. She reports that, "18% of students in the survey who pay rent described keeping up with the payments as a constant struggle, while a further 45% said they struggle from time to time. This, combined, means that over three in five students are struggling to keep up with rent, at least some of the time. "Worryingly, 41% said they have thought about dropping out of university because of either rent or bills. Rent, in particular, is leading a concerning proportion of students to wonder if they can continue with their studies."

Many of these students will have suffered from the chaos and confusion over A levels and GCSE exams during Covid and the utter debacle created by the then Education Secretary Gavin Williams. They need all the help they can get.

The Higher Education Policy Institution and the student housing provider 'Unipol' said that loans should be more accurately described as a "contribution to living costs" to reflect how little they cover.

It really is heart- breaking to see how little the government cares about our future generations.

****

LOOKING A GIFT HORSE IN THE MOUTH

Today (October 30th) there is a letter in the *Times* from the wealthy entrepreneur and philanthropist **Sir James Dyson**. Now I think you will really have to concentrate on this one because it is one of those stories which makes us all feel that yes....it's true.... we have all gone down the rabbit hole.

It is generally believed at the moment that if anything is functioning at all it is because of the many charities we have in this country rather than our non-functioning government. But we also have some rich individuals and some, like Sir Rod Stewart for the NHS and now Sir James Dyson for education, are willing to help out as and when.

Well Dyson wants to give a grant of £6 million to his local state primary school. This will be via his charitable foundation. The school want to build a new science, technology, engineering, arts and mathematics centre as well as seven new classrooms and a school hall. The extra ground is available at no extra cost.

That sounds absolutely wonderful. However.................

Sir James has been trying to give this money since June 2022. But the donation is conditional on the school receiving approval from the Department for Education's regional office to increase the numbers at the school from 420 to 630. And apparently they are saying that if this went ahead the lower-rated surrounding primary schools could be at a risk of closure. As Sir James says they would rather children are bused to out-lying village schools "and deny parents the choice to send their children to this out-standing local school." The head teacher said "It seems crazy that they should look this gift horse in the mouth. Not since Victorian times has someone been this generous to the state sector in primary schools."

The editorial in the *Times* cannot believe the sheer stupidity of this story either and quotes Sunak's meaningless promise to make this country "a global science and technology super –power by 2030".

So there we have it. £6 million for education services rejected by the local DfE.

****

Then today (5th November) Sir James Dyson says in an interview to *The Times* that it is so depressing because nothing ever gets done in Britain today.

Well I think we can all agree with that.

"It's incredibly depressing," he says. "The headmaster, Steve Heal, was bold enough to walk up the road to ask me for the money. I agreed. I'm mystified by the bureaucrats' reluctance to accept. It is a sorry example of how hard it is to get anything done in Britain."

And then: "We need more engineers. When I started in business 30 years ago, we just needed mechanical and electrical engineers. Now we also need software, AI, and battery engineers and we don't educate

58

nearly enough."

He also announced that he is introducing a new master's degree in engineering at the £50 million Dyson Institute, the university which he established seven years ago next to his UK headquarters. Applicants, who will have to have at least two As at A-level, will be paid £22,000 a year, which will almost double over the four-year course. They will not have to take out a student loan. Dyson will fund their tuition to the tune of £250,000 per student.

He believes the government should go back to paying tuition fees. He says most students can't pay back their debts so we are paying for them all anyway.

So here we have millionaire Mr. Sunak laughing and joking with Elon Musk and telling us all to move away from the comfort of a monthly pay packet, become more entrepreneurial and please don't worry if you fail; yet here is one of our most successful entrepreneurs offering a stash of money and the government or local authority turns it down.

Well and truly through the looking glass........or have I said that before?

******

DISAPPEARING TEACHERS

We have a further report about our teachers who continue to be burnt out and to feel undervalued.

There is a disturbing article in the *Observer* today (November 5th) by Julie Henry which says that newly qualified teachers are planning to leave the UK to teach abroad.

Well I think we were aware of the fact that teacher recruitment and retention is at an all-time low. But this is further evidence from the

'National Foundation for Educational Research'.

They report that vacancies posted by schools earlier this year were 93% higher than at the same point in 2019. They also report that the government is missing its teacher-training targets year on year. At primary level, 6,527 applicants were on courses in April this year, down from 8,100 in 2022.

We already know that many children are being taught specialist subjects by non-specialist teachers but this report states that schools are even having to use long-term supply cover to teach classes. This really is unacceptable and is obviously having a severe effect on pupils' attainment standards and is a huge drain on school's budgets.

Ian Hartwright, head of policy for the National Association of Head Teachers, said the longstanding and severe teacher recruitment crisis in England's schools was being acutely felt by those who remain. "The government's chronic underfunding of schools over the last decade has resulted in the loss of teaching assistants and other critical support staff."

Why does the government not hear all of this?

So let us look at where they are all going. Well international schools are booming. And they are very attractive. When I was living in Abu Dhabi I did some supply teaching in the English speaking school there. It was an absolute joy. All resources were available and up- to- date. The pay was good and you were treated as a professional. Everyone was most appreciative including the parents!

So we hear from tutors at the Institute of Education at Manchester University when speaking to MPs who said that "15% of its primary cohort were planning to start careers overseas, with a further 19% still deciding whether to remain in the UK or work abroad, totalling more than 90 teachers."

Other teacher trainers also highlighted the trend: "Potential trainees are interested in more mobile career opportunities, and there is an increased temptation to utilise their qualification, and receive higher salaries and higher professional regard, by teaching abroad," said a group submission, which included Sheffield, King's College London, Cambridge, Bristol and Warwick universities.

And from York university we hear that **"Trainees are asking two key questions: 'Where can I afford to live and work and could I earn more abroad?"**

Well the answer to that last question is a resounding yes. And yes, we need to be very worried. For today, (December 8th) in a report by Nicola Woolcock, education editor of the *Times,* figures from Department for Education reveal that only half as many trainee secondary school teachers have been recruited as are needed in England this year.

****

MENTAL HEALTH

Well we know that the mental health of teachers is suffering inordinately but a report just out (December 2023) from 'Public First' has found that there is a shocking increase in the number of children requiring counselling services for their mental health and that more and more are having to be treated by teachers. They also found that the more that pupils were using school services the more they were pushed down the NHS waiting lists. **'Public First'** is a policy, research, opinion and strategy consultancy. In October 2021, in the midst of the second lockdown, they brought together a coalition of some of the most respected schools in the independent and state sectors calling it 'The Coalition for Youth Mental Health in Schools' to call for radical reform of how mental health is supported in educational settings and their report is shared with the *Times* which comments on it today (13th December).

Of course lockdowns had an extreme effect on our children's mental health. And the report states that this was "not just due to the temporary suspension of co-curricular activity, the sport, music, drama, from which so many of our children derive their sense of self. It was also about the more incidental routines: the chat at registration, the laughter over lunch, the giggling during assembly, the catching up with friends on the bus home, the planning of campaigns or parties, the sharing of concerns or worries, the sheer physical proximity of friends and peers. This is so much more than ephemera for children and teenagers; this is the petri dish for the development of their identity, wholeness and sense of place in the world. The light receded from all of this overnight during Covid and is returning only gradually as the pandemic recedes.

"With all that communal collegiality and everyday connection compromised for so long, it was sadly perhaps inevitable that the mental health of many children, particularly those who were most vulnerable, suffered. Certainly, many schools across the country, are now experiencing unprecedented demand for mental health support and therapeutic services – a demand which mostly can't be satisfied by the current provision, either in schools or beyond them."

Jon Needham, Director of Safeguarding at Oasis Community Learning and vice-chair of the Coalition said "It cannot be for schools alone to fix this problem, it calls for all parts of society, families, local authorities, government, health services and charities to work together to give every young person the support they need, when they need it."

Our teachers are doing a brilliant job at looking after our children as well as actually teaching them and this is just one more burden that they are carrying.

In a joint statement the coalition says that "the state of mental health provision in our country has reached a tipping point."

But again I ask if anyone in government is reading this report? For as Desmond Tutu says:

"There comes a point where we need to stop just pulling people out of the river. We need to go upstream and find out why they're falling in."

****

BLUE SKIES?

The entire education system in the UK needs to be overhauled and the Ofsted approach to the inspection of schools needs to be changed in line with it. The present system is creaking at the seams and the future requires an up-dated, fully funded, innovative, modern and forward-looking curriculum. The Times Education Commission was published last year and was a brilliant report by many educational experts. The commission's report was welcomed by Sir Tony Blair, Sir John Major and Bridget Phillipson (shadow secretary for Education) along with ten former education secretaries. So has the government listened?

Here are the main points so you can judge for yourselves.

They highlight 12 points:

A British Baccalaureate instead of the narrow A level system.

Well I think this **has** been mentioned by the PM. This is a good start, you might think, but sadly I don't see even a glimmer of recognition in any of the following as the words in this chapter would indicate.

Electives Premium to be granted to all schools to be spent on drama, music, dance, sport and a National Citizen Service consisting of volunteering and outdoor expeditions for every pupil.

A new cadre of career academies with links to industry and a focus on creativity and entrepreneurialism.

Help for early years with a boost for funding and when every child would have a unique pupil number from birth and every primary school would have a library.

A tutorial boost when undergraduates could act as tutors and earn credits towards their degrees.

Digital skills which would give every child a laptop or tablet.

Welcome Wellbeing which should be at the heart of education with a counsellor in every school to encourage pupils to actively build resilience.

Restore the status of teachers with better career development and a new category of consultant teachers.

A reformed Ofsted with a wider range of metrics including wellbeing, and school culture.

Special needs focus to give a greater focus on inclusion and training for teachers to be able to identify needs.

50 new university campuses and a transferable credit system between universities and colleges.

A 15 year strategy putting education above short term party politics.

And just to remind you why we need this as if you didn't know.

Between 2010 and 2025 spending on the health service will have increased by 42% whilst the education budget will have gone up by 3% over the same period.

So there we have it. It's been done. It is all there and it is amazing. All the details can be found on the *Times'* website.

****

BACK TO REALITY

But of course this is language not associated with the Conservative party in power today.

In fact I see a sentence in a *Guardian* article by Zoe Williams written in June 2021 when she says that **"Since 2010, the cuts affecting children have been so swingeing and so wide-ranging, so short-sighted and so interconnected, as to often look like deliberate acts of cruelty."**

Then I see the House of Commons Committee report, with recommendations to government.

This is the Fifty-Fifth Report of Session 2022–23 Education recovery in schools in England, published on the 7th June 2023.

I just quote some of their conclusions and recommendations.

They say "It is alarming that it may take a decade for the gap in attainment between disadvantaged pupils and others to return to what it was before the COVID-19 pandemic.

The Department should publish a plan setting out how, building on good practice, it will reduce the disadvantage gap as quickly as possible, and the expected trajectory.

"Effective recovery relies on pupils being at school but absence is higher than it was before the COVID-19 pandemic, particularly among disadvantaged pupils.

"We share the Department's disappointment that 13% of schools did not take up the National Tutoring Programme in 2021/22, meaning pupils at these schools missed out on the benefits of subsidised tutoring.

"We are not confident that schools will be able to afford to provide tutoring on the scale required to support all the pupils who need

it once the Department withdraws its subsidy.

"The Department has no interim targets to track progress towards the 2030 attainment ambitions set out in the Schools White Paper.

"The Department pointed us to the performance metrics that it published every year in its Outcome Delivery Plan. It said that it published a wide range of metrics at Key Stages 2 and 4, and the results of Key Stage 1 tests such as the phonics screening check. The Department assured us that it used all of these measures to hold itself to account, and that it expected other people to use them to hold it to account for progress. We note, however, that the Department's most recent Outcome Delivery Plan was published in July 2021, nearly two years ago."

So here is the final paragraph of the report by the government published on the 24th September 2023.

"Statistics on attainment in KS1, KS2 and phonics at regional and local authority level and broken down by pupil and school characteristics will be published in Autumn 2023. This will provide the department with the latest picture of progress towards the 2030 ambitions on attainment. Detailed 2023 attainment data across key stage 2 and key stage 4 will not be available prior to the 2023 summer parliamentary recess. Key stage 2 national statistics were released on 11 July 2023. This shows that overall, more pupils met the expected standard in this year's mathematics and writing assessments than last year, and although reading has declined from last year it remains consistent with results in 2019 prior to the pandemic. The department continues to use evidence and wider insights to review progress towards our 2030 ambitions, across different cohorts and phases, to determine how best to support all pupils, including those who are disadvantaged."

Here is part of what they say about the results of the phonics tests on their autumn statement published on the 12th October 2023 on GOV.UK

"In 2023, 79% of pupils met the expected standard in year 1, up from 75% in 2022. Previously, the proportion of pupils who met the standard in year 1 increased year-on-year from 58% in 2012 to 82% in 2018, remained stable at 82% in 2019, then decreased to 75% in 2022."

Well I think that is some improvement but not yet "consistent with results in 2019" pre Covid levels. Certainly more work to be done and Mr. Sunak should not be boasting about our brilliant phonics results at PMQs.

****

As schools struggle to survive in porta cabins I hear today (11th November) from the 'Good Law Project.' They say:-

"We can reveal that a firm owned by a Conservative Party donor has bagged an £11.5m Government contract to supply temporary classrooms for schools built with unsafe concrete. The Department of Education has asked Wernick Buildings Limited to provide "temporary accommodation and associated services to mitigate schools disruption due to rebuilding, condition and refurbishment programmes". The company is controlled by David Wernick, who has given more than £71,000 to the Tories either through his companies or in a personal capacity between 2001 and 2021. More than half this amount – £42,000 – has been donated since 2019.

"Our latest investigation with the *Daily Mirror* has sparked calls in Parliament for the Education Secretary, Gillian Keegan, to come to the House of Commons to explain why this multi-million pound contract has been handed to a Tory donor's firm."

Thank you 'Good Law Project' for exposing this. We need to know. And we need to hear from the Education Secretary.

****

I also see this today about the failings of provision for **children with special educational needs and disabilities** (SEND) in Hertfordshire. Ofsted and the Care Quality Commission service found that this service in Hertfordshire received the lowest rating possible, with some children found to have been waiting for more than 78 weeks for help.

The inspection, completed over four days in July, found the rate of exclusions for children and young people with care plans was a "concern". They said that, "A significant number of parents feel they have no alternative but to educate their child at home while they are waiting for a place in a special school to become available."

So yet another reason for children to be absent from school.

Hertfordshire County Council and the NHS Hertfordshire and West Essex Integrated Care Board are part of the local area partnership responsible for planning and commissioning SEND services.

It has been given 35 days to publish a "priority action plan" and a monitoring inspection will be carried out within 18 months.

The partnership said: "We want to say sorry to you, our families. We understand the scale of the issues and know that too many children and young people with SEND and their families have not had the service and outcomes they need and deserve.

We have already put in place strong improvement plans."

Actually I don't think so. In fact the entire country is facing a shortage of SEND teachers due to the UK's complete lack of specialist SEND teacher training – it's not even part of the PGCE or BA qualifications. And in England, almost 1.5 million pupils need SEND support. One senior teacher was visibly upset as she explained to the mother of an autistic boy that even if she could afford to pay for a special teacher, which she couldn't, there were none anywhere to be found. This is at a time when schools are having to make teachers redundant as their budgets run out. This is leading to larger classes and more stressed staff leaving. As they leave they are not being replaced.

I run out of appropriate words and have to just leave this hanging there for you to see and absorb and despair.

****

CHARITIES FOR CHILDREN

But now I have to report something that will really cheer us up. I think we need it.

It is about a charity (again) called **'Go Beyond'.**

This is one of their values on their website.

"We put children at the centre of our charity, make them our priority, involve them in shaping our work, listen to their voices."

I **LOVE** them already.

They are based in **Cornwall and the Peak District** and basically they give disadvantaged children a wonderful free break "under wide open skies" for a week in the countryside.

They will get referrals from any individual working with young people in a professional capacity and offer this amazing experience.

They say that "Go Beyond's expert staff and committed volunteers give children and young people who have been bereaved, abused or bullied, who are living in poverty or caring for loved ones the chance to escape their worries and pressures."

I am getting very emotional just reading about this because it is so different from nearly everything else that I have been writing about. It is wonderful and just what so many of our young people need.

As I said it is a charity and so relies totally on charitable giving.

These are some of the activities they offer children from 8 to 15.

Horse riding, rock climbing, surfing, baking and toasting marshmallows around the campfire. As they say "don't let anyone tell you that's not a real activity".

There are ball games, trampolines and giant Jenga and movie nights and board games. They also have an 'Arts and Crafts Barn' where they say "your imagination can go wild making, creating and drawing AND a Games Room with football tables, table tennis and pool."

Wellies and rain coats are provided as one of the favourite occupations is splashing in puddles. And of course there are the stepping stones in Dovedale over the River Dove. I remember hopping over them as a very young child. I thought it was brilliant.

It is a mobile phone free week but if anyone is homesick they can arrange for them to speak to someone from home.

There is a maximum of 16 children, 8 girls and 8 boys at each centre.

They say that "No child is ever forced to take part in anything they do not want to do and activities do vary slightly according to the time of the year, weather and age of the children. Our hope is for every child to go home believing in themselves and knowing they can achieve more than they ever thought possible."

Oh my goodness. These people are my heroes and I hope they are yours too. It is only because I have just spent a few days in the Peak District and read an article that I homed in on them.

****

Wow, I have just discovered yet another amazing charity doing the government's work for them. This one is called 'Magic Breakfast, fuel for learning.'

Well we all know how the present government refuses to provide children with free school meals whilst happily eating subsidised three-course meals in the House of Commons. We also know how children arrive at school having had nothing to eat and how this affects their behaviour.

Well 'Magic Breakfast' is a charity that delivers free breakfasts to school children facing hunger every day. Why have I never heard of them before?

On their website they say that, "We work in schools working within high levels of disadvantage, helping head teachers target the children most in need without making those children stand out or feel embarrassed. We believe that breakfast provision should always be stigma-free and open to all."

The Food Foundation says that by September 2022 4 million children in the UK were at risk of hunger. With the present cost of living crisis more and more children are going hungry.

'Magic Breakfast' will look at all applications from head teachers as they ask them:

"Do you have children arriving at school without having eaten breakfast? Are you noticing the effects of hunger in the classroom? Do you want to ensure every pupil has the right fuel for learning? We are happy to consider applications from schools in the UK for our healthy breakfast provision and expert support."

They will hold their details on file and contact them as soon as funding becomes available. **For a school in England to be eligible**, at least 35% of pupils should be recorded as eligible for Pupil Premium. I just quote a little of the views of one head teacher, Catherine Jones, head teacher at one of their long-standing partner schools, Thorney Close Primary School in Sunderland.

She says that:

"One of the biggest changes in our school is the children now arrive on time, and attendance has got better. The beginning of the day is so calm and focused, and it's made a massive difference on learning because the children are now all fed and ready to learn.

Another huge difference is that we no longer have children who are masking hunger. If anybody is still hungry after breakfast, they're not frightened to ask for something else.

'Magic Breakfast' has enabled us to reach out to every child in the school, it's really important no child gets missed. The children are all happy because they've had something to eat as well as social time, and the parents are less stressed because they aren't worrying about getting the children ready and feeding them before school.

"So it's just really strengthened the bond that we have with the children and the families. It's become part of our culture here at Thorney Close. When we started classroom breakfasts up again after lockdown the children were just so excited, because for them it was also about getting back to normality again."

They can manage to do this with money given by public-spirited and generous people.

Why can't the government do it with our taxes?

****

BUILDING MAINTENANCE

And today 19th November a report is published by the 'Committee of Public Accounts' which is absolutely damning on the lack of progress by the DfE pertaining to the building maintenance programme.

We all know about the appalling state of our schools in general and we now all know about the RAAC concrete but this report also highlights the **danger of asbestos in schools**. But it is the complete absence of concern or urgency by the Education Department which is now so shocking. This report is to be found on the UK Parliament web- site and so is available for all to see. They make 10 recommendations which fully display the incompetence and criminal negligence of this government. They are as follows:

1. **DfE still has incomplete knowledge on the number and condition of schools with RAAC, with questions about the reliability of some of its information.**

2. **DfE's risk appetite regarding the school estate, and how this aligns with its recent approach on RAAC, appears unclear.**

3. **Schools are uncertain about the support they can access to mitigate RAAC-related issues, and how they will be reimbursed financially.**

4. **There remains a lack of transparency for schools, parents and communities on where RAAC exists and how long it will take to be fixed.**

5. **DfE has incomplete knowledge of the prevalence of asbestos across the school estate.**

6. **Unacceptable numbers of pupils are learning in poorly maintained or potentially unsafe buildings.**

7. **DfE has focused on reactive measures addressing immediate building concerns that often fail to take account of longer-term value for money considerations.**

8. **The School Rebuilding Programme is behind its initial schedule for getting contracts in place and schools built.**

9. There is considerable variation across the school estate, including regional disparity in the condition of school buildings and differences in school types and governance models, which will influence the type of support DfE needs to provide.

10. It is unclear whether decisions concerned with addressing the condition of the estate are coordinated with those relating to the need for school places.

They go on to say that the state of disrepair of some schools is so bad that 700,000 pupils are learning in classrooms that need a major rebuild or refurbishment and that they are learning in "poorly maintained or potentially unsafe buildings."

Paul Whiteman, general secretary of the NAHT school leaders' union, said it "beggars belief" that ministers still lacked a clear plan to deal with deteriorating school buildings. "We urgently need clarity from ministers on when RAAC will be dealt with and a proper long-term plan to ensure the school estate is fit for purpose, both backed by the significant new funding that will be needed. This should be a top priority for next week's autumn statement."

Well we will listen very carefully to that autumn statement.

But the other problem which is so frightening is the presence of asbestos in so many schools. And the DfE does not seem to know which schools are affected. But it is a fact that all companies who own buildings or who have built them for leasing out have been required by law to maintain an asbestos register for every building for years. Yes asbestos is safe while undisturbed and this is the government's defence when last year the Work and Pensions committee recommended the government establish a national register of schools with asbestos. The government declined, insisting asbestos was safer left in place. But if, for example, a classroom ceiling collapses, or a school is refurbished or partially demolished to remove RAAC, it can release fibres that, if inhaled, can prove fatal.

And according to data from the Health and Safety Executive, **around 11 teachers or ex-teachers have died from asbestos-related conditions, each year, since 2011.**

If there is nothing at all about the state of the infrastructure of our schools in the Chancellor's statement next week we have to be prepared for a continuation of a shocking lack of interest in the welfare of our children.

****

November 22nd. Well there is absolutely nothing for education in the Chancellor's budget. Head teachers have called the government's failure to invest in school staff and crumbling buildings in the autumn statement "an absolute disgrace".

****

DISABILITY RIGHTS

But I get an email from openDemocracy today (23rd November) from Dr.China Mills who is the Disability Justice Lead for '**Healing Justice London**.' She manages their 'Deaths by Welfare Project', exploring how welfare policies harm people and what can be learned from the strategies of disabled people and bereaved families in fighting for justice. She is Senior Lecturer at City, University of London where she researches and teaches global mental health with a focus on state and corporate production of harm, distress and deaths by suicide.

But as I read this email I am shocked. She, together with John Pring, have been studying the effect on disabled people by the Department for Work and Pensions (DWP) since 2021 **"showing the links between welfare policy and disabled people's deaths."**

Now this is a book about children but I think it is important to know how the government treats disabled adults as this will often affect children and this is very concerning.

Ms. Mills slates the autumn budget proposals to cut benefits and writes "The welfare system has taken another hit today via a 'benefits crackdown' in Jeremy Hunt's autumn statement. Since the 'welfare reform' of 2007, disabled people have been on the receiving end of these dehumanising and punishing policies that make people out as 'undeserving', prioritise work over people, and make life unlivable.

"But we now have evidence the Department for Work and Pensions (DPW) knows its policies kill people.

It has been repeatedly warned of this fact and has even confirmed it in its own research. It took years of campaigning by disabled people to uncover this evidence, which largely comes in the form of DWP reviews into deaths of claimants.

Now it has been brought together as part of the 'Deaths by Welfare' project at 'Healing Justice London'. On its website it states that: "Our 'Deaths by Welfare' Project investigates deaths linked to welfare reform and the violence of state austerity. The aim of the project is to make visible the slow and bureaucratic violence of the State, and to contextualise welfare related deaths as issues of disability, spatial, racial and economic justice. Integral to this work is honouring, uplifting and learning from disabled people's lived experience and resistance."

'The Equality and Human Rights Monitor report', published today, is supposed to assess the status of equality and human rights across Britain since 2018. But it is being heavily criticised over its unwillingness to hold the government to account over its repeated breaches of disabled people's rights.

Now most of this report is focused on adults but there is a short piece about education.

It has always been the policy in education to be inclusive as much as possible with disabled children being educated, with support, in mainstream schools. So this is rather surprising. The DNS says "The report appears to welcome funding that allowed the opening of a string of new special schools, with provision for up to 3,000 disabled pupils, without pointing out that the UN committee on the rights of persons with disabilities has criticised the UK government for the 'persistence of a dual education system' that segregates increasing numbers of disabled children in special schools.

The **report also fails to point out that article 24 of the UN disability convention** requires the development of a fully inclusive education system."

Why are they doing this? Long term evidence has always said that students with **disability** who go to mainstream schools are more likely to enrol in post-secondary education, to be employed and to be able to live independently. According to one research review, students in mainstream schools also tend to have better social skills.

Disability and education advocates argue special schools are a form of segregation and go against students' human rights. Even the language skills of pre-schoolers with disabilities improve when they can interact with their peers without disability in the same classroom.

I repeat: why are they spending all this money on something which is not beneficial to the education of disabled children?

****

It is so important for those who are responsible in any way for the welfare of our children to fully understand them. I find it very distressing when I see examples of children being punished for acting like children. I was a primary school teacher and believe me when I say that I know how disruptive some children can be. But many schools are now academies. Academies receive funding directly from the government and are run by an academy trust. Academies have more control over how they do things, for example they do not have to follow the national curriculum and can set their own term dates. This can of course be liberating and can produce some inspirational ideas. They are all subject to Ofsted inspections but I just feel that they do need close scrutiny at all times.

For example I do find the following very worrying.

Anna Fazackerley and Michael Savage of the *Observer* have analysed the latest **DofE annual data on suspensions and exclusions in academy schools** and found that in some of the strictest schools they had suspension rates which far exceeded the national average in the year 2021 -2022. Two of the country's biggest trusts, Astrea and Outward Grange Academies Trust had schools with a suspension rate of about 200% of their pupil numbers compared with the national average of 6.9%. Mind you they said that this could be due to the fact that some students had been suspended many times.

Really? If that is the case have they never sat down and thought that perhaps suspension is not actually working?

And what of the dreadful behaviour which is cause for suspension? Well obviously persistent aggressive or violent behaviour has to be stopped in its tracks but so-called 'disruptive behaviour' can apparently consist of not having a pencil to not taking off your jacket. Some school academies have 'zero tolerance' systems whereby children are not allowed to speak in corridors or in the classroom unless given permission to speak.

For goodness sake children are naturally noisy, curious and full of energy and this needs to be channelled into positive outcomes not stifled. Very often suspension is the lazy answer to a problem by teachers not prepared to give enough time and thought to children in these academy schools.

Anne Longfield, former Children's Commissioner, warned that poorer children and those with special educational needs were more likely to be suspended or excluded. She said: "Young people who end up being excluded are vulnerable to being exploited by criminal gangs and their life chances are diminished."

Yes it is always the disadvantaged who suffer the most.

****

Then there is a Christmas message for all our children who go to state schools. A report in the *Observer* by Anna Fazackerley states that there are now 231 schools and colleges with RAAC, according to the latest government figures released earlier this month. The *Observer* has been told that the Department for Education is refusing to commit to funding or even give any timescales for starting work, with building experts estimating that schools will be waiting years for new safe buildings.

The head teacher of a primary school in the north of England with confirmed RAAC in its roof, who spoke to the *Observer* on condition of anonymity, said: "I can't get any information. There is no indication of when they will decide, never mind a decision."

After weeks of pushing, the head has managed to secure funding from the DfE for temporary scaffolding that will ensure the school's roof doesn't collapse, but he still has no idea whether the government will choose to demolish the whole school, which is in a "very bad state" generally, or whether it will just be given a new roof.

An education consultant who works closely with the DfE but asked not to be named to protect the schools he is advising, described the government's response as "a shambles". In one primary school the children have to cross a car park to get from one part of the school to another as the central part of the school building is unsafe. Would you be happy with that?

2026 is the earliest date given for any possible repair work to be completed anywhere. And that will only happen if work is started now and continues "at pace". Well, as we have seen, the words "at pace" do not belong in the vocabulary of the present government.

And the government is refusing to give any extra help to pupils doing exams who have not had access to science labs or design and technology work rooms because they are closed due to RAAC. Some children have had to switch courses because they are unable to do the required experiments and head teachers have asked for them to be given special consideration. But no........the Department for Education said no and that it was "not possible to make changes to exams and assessments for only some groups of students".

****

26TH DECEMBER 2023

The title of this book is 'Our Lost Children'. Most of the children I write about are ignored and un-cared for.

But on the 21st October, 1966 116 children were lost for ever, together with five teachers. On a mountain slope above the village of Aberfan near Merthyr Tydfil in South Wales a colliery coal slag heap came crashing down the mountain at a speed of more than 80 miles an hour. Children had just arrived at Pantglas Junior School and were about to start lessons after assembly when 1.4 million cubic feet of slurry came crashing against the walls of the building suffocating nearly everyone inside. Anyone who saw, as I did, the images on television of frantic parents scrabbling at the rubble with their bare hands to look for their children will never forget it.

The National Coal Board had previously had complaints from residents about the apparent dangers of coal slurry being tipped at the rear of the school. They had corresponded with the County Borough Council between July 1963 and March 1964.

Meetings were held between the council and the NCB in 1965 when it was agreed that the clogged piped and drainage ditches, which were the cause of severe flooding, would be fixed. No action had been taken by October 1966 when the tip collapsed.

So why am I mentioning this now?

Because I read an article in the *Guardian,* by Steven Morris. It is shocking. The Labour –led Welsh government has published maps which show 350 disused coal tips near to villages and small communities which they say are a threat. They fear that any of them could cause a landslip.

Edmund Richards, aged 80, who worked for 40 years as a miner told the *Guardian* that, "They're on the move, No doubt. From time to time, inspectors will come and have a look, and say all is fine, but everyone around here knows they are on the move, on the slide."

It is often difficult to spot them because they are covered in scrub and trees but Mr. Edmunds says that "everyone who lives nearby knows where they are and is worried about them. They need to get on and sort them out once and for all. **It's only a matter of time before something terrible happens."**

Of those more hazardous ones, 79 are in Rhondda Cynon Taf, 59 in Merthyr Tydfil, and 51 in Caerphilly.

So what are those in government doing about this? Well absolutely nothing.

Actually that is not quite true. They are passing the buck. Westminster Conservative government says it's nothing to do with them but the devolved Labour Welsh government say they can't afford the £50m a year for 10 to 15 years that it would take to fix them all. The UK government say that the Welsh were given the largest annual settlement in the history of devolution at the spending review in 2021.

The Welsh say that the whole of the UK benefitted from the coal so they should be responsible for clearing it all up.

I say please, please stop this ridiculous conversation and both governments work together for the safety of our children and their families. Surely you can get around a table and decide who can afford to pay for what. Or is that too much to expect?

****

Schools are supposed to be safe places for all of our children. There is so much work to be done........ practically, economically and compassionately.

****

"No other investment yields as great a return
as the investment in education.
An educated workforce
is the foundation of every community
and the future of every economy."

Brad Henry.
American lawyer and politician

****

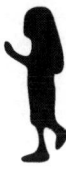

CHILDREN'S CARE HOMES

It is up to local authorities to find suitable residential accommodation for vulnerable children. Indeed they have a legal duty to find secure, safe, local accommodation to meet the needs of the children they look after. But too many children are being sent miles from home because of a shortage of placements and in today's climate finding any suitable accommodation is proving to be extremely difficult and very expensive. Ofsted found that about 30 children are being placed in Scottish secure units at any one time due to a shortage of places in England.

Private providers of children's homes and foster care are making "significant and persistent" profits by charging cash-strapped local authorities elevated prices for increasingly scarce placements, the 'Competition and Markets Authority' has said. The largest private providers of children's homes are now charging councils an average of £3,830 a week per child, with an average operating profit margin of 23%, according to the CMA's interim report on children's social care.

As at 31st March 2023, private companies ran 85% of children's homes providing 81% of places whilst Local Authorities ran 12% of children's homes, providing 14% of places

I have been reading many reports on this issue and all of them are extremely concerning.

Most of these reports have been sent to the government and we hear of various agendas and promises but since the reshuffle in August 2023 children's social care now has its fifth minister in two years.

David Johnston MP is the new Parliamentary Under-Secretary of State for Children, Families and Wellbeing. The British Association of Social Workers England raised concerns about the turnover of children's ministers.

While wishing David Johnston well, BASW England said his appointment "sadly sends a message that a sustainable and consistent ministerial approach to children, their families and wellbeing is not a political priority for this government". It went on to say that "At a time of major upheaval and reform in children's social care in England, we desperately need a leadership that is focused on the needs of children and families, not political ambitions. The fact that Johnston is the fifth minister to take on this role in two years should worry all of us who want to see stability and support that is too often denied to the very children the minister seeks to represent."

But the government has set up 'The **Children's Social Care National Framework'. This** is a government consultation on principles for practice, expected outcomes, and indicators for children's social care. The framework was launched on February 2nd, 2023, and the consultation period ended on May 11th, 2023. So this is something for Mr. Johnston to get out of his in-tray as quickly as possible. The framework aims to provide a shared understanding of the expectations for all those who are working to ensure that children, young people, and families, whatever their circumstances, can thrive.

However, it is too early (October 2023) to say whether the framework is working in practice as it was launched so recently and the implementation period is still ongoing. The government has said that it will release the National Framework and Dashboard indicators by the end of the year.

Josh MacAlister who is chairing the independent review of children's social care in England, said the report showed the market was broken and failing too many children.

So I see the National Framework indicators published in December 2023. It is 60 pages long and it is full of very fine words and recommendations. You couldn't ask for anything more. Except, well, maybe you could. There were, so far as I could see, two things missing. There was no mention of where the extra funding was going to come from and nothing about where the extra staff were going to come from. Both are vital I would have thought.

****

But I go back to a report by the Children's Commissioner on 'Private Provision in Children's Social Care' published in November 2020 when a number of points were raised and I quote them as follows.

"Since 2016 there have been a number of mergers and acquisitions that involved a large number of homes, carers or residential schools changing hands at the same time. If a provider changes hands it is usually because the purchaser believes they can obtain greater profit from it in future. Conversations with staff who have worked at children's homes before and after a takeover paint a complicated picture of what this process means for them and for children. In some homes that were taken over, spending on children was reduced after acquisition. One staff member said that the activity budget for children had been cut to an amount that "doesn't go very far". Another said they had to fight to persuade the new company to keep personal savings accounts for the children, despite this being a statutory right for looked after children."

There is concern that "not enough information is made available about the way care is commissioned and provided by independent companies, and that not enough resources are dedicated to oversight of the sector. Straightforward answers on profit, ownership, debt and costs are not available, as private companies have expanded to fill a niche left by local authorities, as opposed to being brought in as part of a coordinated strategy. More work, underpinned by better data and improved transparency, is required in order to produce more definitive answers to these questions, and ensure that children are getting the best care – and the taxpayer value for money."

The problems with children's social care are enormous.

Anne Longfield, the former Children's Commissioner for England has said that the most vulnerable children are being "failed by the state" and a broken residential care system. "The system has been allowed to slip deeper into crisis," she said and "greater use of private provision has led to a fragmented, uncoordinated and irrational system amid "significant profits".

Ms. Longfield has published three reports detailing the plight of children the system "doesn't know what to do with".

She said the government has failed to respond to previous warnings that thousands of these children are in danger of becoming victims of criminal and sexual exploitation.

Older children were found to be living in "disgusting" conditions akin to a prison cell, one of the reports said.

It described how one 17-year-old said her accommodation was filthy and smelly, with just one working shower - covered in mould - between 14 children and young adults.

"Elsewhere children have told us they have not even been provided with the means to eat or sleep - things like duvet covers, plates or cutlery," the same report said.

Some of the stories we hear from children in some of these very expensive profit making homes are heart -breaking and shocking. They talk to investigations as do some staff who have left these homes in disgust.

****

A report by Noel Titheradge of BBC news in June 2022 makes shocking reading. We hear of two specific companies, the Calcot Services for Children and the Hesley run homes.

'**Calcot Services for Children**' which runs eight homes, four schools and supported living accommodation in southern England made profits of 42% in 2020 and 36% in 2021, using an industry-standard measure.

That is more than double the average annual profit made by the biggest 15 providers of children's services in Great Britain over the past five years - as highlighted in a recent report by the government>s competition watchdog.

The BBC has seen leaked company records and confidential local authority briefings. It has also spoken to a dozen current and former Calcot employees.

Their investigation found:

- Children had reported being groomed for sex, given alcohol, and also assaulted by staff.

- Allegations of child-on-child sexual abuse and suicide attempts after youngsters had absconded were not reported to Ofsted despite an obligation to do so.

- Calcot did not provide some dedicated care and teaching staff despite receiving specific funding from local authorities.

- Claims of inadequate staffing at homes where there were serious incidents - including an assault and rape allegation.

- Some support workers had been asked to sign non-disclosure agreements when they left the company.

The present Children's Commissioner for England, Dame Rachel de Souza, said she was "appalled" by these findings and said they revealed "actual harm".

She is "concerned" that there is no mechanism to immediately flag a provider over serious safeguarding incidents and the sector as a whole included some "exceptional" private children's homes, but unfortunately "some of the worst providers" were also harboured by the industry."

She said it seemed wrong that some providers were "still allowed to make large profits".

"The entire system needs radical reform."

Then we see that there has been a follow-up report by the 'Child Safeguarding Practice Review Panel' and its recommendations follow its earlier report on the systematic abuse and neglect of more than 100 young people at three facilities in Doncaster run by the **'Hesley Group'**.

That inquiry identified a "culture of abuse" in which children were physically, sexually and emotionally harmed by staff over a number of years. The panel described the lengthy catalogue of abuse as "dreadful and harrowing".

The children subjected to abuse in the 'Hesley'-run homes are described by the report as some of society's most vulnerable, typically with learning disabilities, autism and complex health needs.

Although the authorities in South Yorkshire finally launched an investigation into the abuse in March 2021, the latest panel report revealed that regulator Ofsted had failed to intervene for more than three years despite hundreds of complaints, serious incident notifications and staff whistleblowing reports about conditions at the three homes.

Children were punched, kicked, verbally taunted and subjected to inappropriate restraint, including being locked up overnight in bathrooms. The reports of cruelty and abuse at the homes are subject to a criminal investigation by South Yorkshire police.

Black female children placed at the Doncaster homes routinely had their hair shaved short when they arrived at times against the wishes of their parents, the panel report said, describing it as an "unacceptable practice that was both de-personalising and degrading for the children".

The panel chair, Annie Hudson, urged ministers to "honour and provide some measure of justice" to the abused children. "This will require unequivocal political and professional will, along with necessary investment, to deliver the substantive and strategic long-term changes that will make a difference to children's lives," she said.

Education secretary Gillian Keegan said she was horrified by the abuse and failings at the three Doncaster homes. That, I believe, is her total response.

According to a BBC investigation earlier this year, local authorities paid about £250,000 a year to place a child at the Doncaster homes, contributing to millions in profits for the 'Hesley Group'. Last year the competition watchdog said the "dysfunctional" children's residential care market in England meant councils paid excessive fees for often substandard services.

Many of the children at the three Doncaster facilities could have been supported at home, the panel said, but with councils finding it "difficult to invest in the range of community provision required" they often had little option but to place children in expensive homes far away where they risked being "out of sight and out of mind".

John Pearce, president of the Association of Directors of Children's Services, said: "The impact that 13 years of austerity has had on our ability to offer the kind of local solutions that allow all children to remain in provision close to home and connected to their communities, wherever possible, cannot be understated."

As we hear that the number of children in care in England could reach almost 100,000 by 2025, it is worrying to note that councils with social care responsibilities in England are facing a £2.1bn funding shortfall next year, according to research from the public sector workers' union, Unison.

They said that the black hole local authorities face in 2022-23 will lead to "huge service and staff cuts", unless central government steps in to increase funding.

Taking a child into care is the most serious and expensive decision a local authority has to make.

In 2015, 69,000 children in England were looked after by councils - but by March 2020, the figure was 80,080.

'The Howard League for Penal Reform' reports that:-

- 'Looked after' children living in children's homes are being criminalised at excessively high rates compared to all other groups of children, including those in other types of care.

- Staff in children's homes are too frequently calling out the police, often over minor incidents.

- Exposure to the criminal justice system affects the already damaged life chances of these highly vulnerable children.

- Three-quarters of England's 1,760 children's homes are run by private companies.

- Lack of transparency, particularly in relation to private children's homes, means that homes are not accountable, bad practices are hidden and children suffer.

- These problems are widely recognised by the government, the police, local authorities, Ofsted and other relevant authorities but they are not being addressed.

- In 2014, 5,220 children were living in children's homes. The number of children going into care is at its highest point in 30 years.

****

Then there is the problem of secure children's homes.

These homes are licensed to deprive young people of their liberty when referred by the courts. Young people placed in these homes are either sentenced or on remand through the justice system or placed due to local authority concerns that a young person is a serious risk to themselves or others.

At present these homes lack sufficient capacity to provide a place for all young people referred to them for welfare reasons. When this happens local authorities must provide an alternative accommodation that meets the young person's needs and keeps them safe.

But children are having to wait for an unacceptable amount of time before they can be placed in a home. According to figures obtained from the Department for Education after a freedom of information request, the average time a child who has been deprived of their liberty for their own protection will spend waiting for a secure placement is currently 65 days.

In July 2022 data from Ofsted showed that about 50 children were waiting for a place each day, up from 25 the year before.

Kathy Evans, the chief executive of the charity 'Children England', which represents the voluntary sector on children and family issues said: "This is a long-term abject commissioning failure. Children have been dying for lack of suitable care since the start of my career in

1993 and they're still dying now. There have been no serious strategic attempts to commission secure children's homes for welfare, as opposed to custodial, reasons, in three decades."

Some children are never able to live in registered, regulated secure homes at all, but are instead placed in unregistered and therefore unlawful ones.

Carolyne Willow, the director of children's charity 'Article 39', said: "Family court judges have been sending their judgments to the education secretary, the children's commissioner and the chief social worker, yet this still hasn't registered as a national child protection emergency."

Ms. Willow has been appealing since June 2020 against a refusal by the DfE to answer her freedom of information request for sight of a report about children dying and suffering other serious harms whilst in local authority care.

The' National Statutory Body for Child Safeguarding' has refused to publish a report which analysed 48 separate incidents where children in care died or were seriously harmed.

But Ms. Willow says that: "Depriving children of their liberty is a grave measure which invariably exposes systematic failures in care, protection and support over many years. **We need the whole of government to accept its obligations towards children in the care of the state, which is why we are pressing for legal duties that would guarantee sufficient funding for councils and effective national planning."**

****

CHILDREN AGED 16-18

Ministers banned the placing of children under the age of 16 in unregulated accommodation but there is serious concern about the fact that children between the ages 16-18 are often placed in unregulated homes.

A report was commissioned by the 'Child Safeguarding Practice Review Panel' and their annual report, published May 2021 states that:-

"Children aged 16 and 17 who are in care and live in unregulated accommodation do not receive day-to-day care, and there is no consistent adult supervision. Children must take full responsibility for their finances and their health, including hospital appointments. The Competition and Markets Authority has reported that this type of accommodation reaps the highest rate of profit within the children's care system, with the 15 largest providers making on average £330 per week profit (35.5%) per child."

I ask you to look at your 16/17 year old child, grand- child, nephew or niece and ask yourself whether they could survive completely on their own if they had been suffering from severe mental or physical trauma.

For just today, October 24th 2023, the information Ms. Willow has been fighting for has been released as she has won a legal challenge to gain access to it.

It is no wonder that the government has been trying to keep this a secret. This nine page report looked at 89 instances of death or serious harm among vulnerable young people between the aged of 16 and 18 over the two years to June 2020.

So many children, for that is who they are, were put into unregulated accommodation without any residential staff. The report found that a "high number of vulnerable females" were victims of rape, sexual assault or child sexual exploitation, and boys in care were victims of stabbing or assaults.

Ms. Willow said, "**There are children taking their own lives, being raped and sexually assaulted, stabbed and beaten up and found dead on roads and rail tracks. These were all children for whom the state was responsible – being in care was meant to protect them and to help them recover from past abuse and trauma. Yet they suffered in the most appalling way.**"

Well the answer from the Department for Education to this devastating critique is to say that these homes will be inspected now every three years (three years????) and of course loads of money is being poured in which is the standard answer by this government to all criticism about anything.

Has there ever been a more misleading name than "Children's Care Homes? In my previous books I refer to these homes as "We Don't Care Homes".

Make no mistake, children are being mistreated and abused and tortured at the hands of the state. I am shocked and I am sure that you are too.

****

And today (30th October) we read this. 'The Institute for Government' is a leading government think tank. It has just produced its annual report on the state of public services and it says that they are "crumbling" and face a state of "perpetual" crisis.

Well yes I think we are all aware of that.

They go on to say that these "dire" public services were performing worse than they did before Covid – and much worse than when the Conservatives came to power in 2010. And to complete their criticism of this government they tell us something else that we all know which is that the government's refusal to negotiate on public sector pay for months had extended the duration of strikes and brought more disruption. "Escaping this will not be easy and whoever forms the next government will be hindered by the short- sighted decisions of its predecessors," they say. **But then it predicted that children's social care would be performing worse in 2027-28 than on the eve of the pandemic.** The report covered several public services including hospitals, GPs, the police, courts, prisons, adult social care, schools and children's social care. Most of these of course will impact on the well-being of children in one way or another.

I continue to be horrified at the lack of concern by those responsible for the welfare of our children. The fact that they think it is OK to inspect some of these homes only once every three years says it all.

****

DECEMBER 2023, CHILD CRUELTY

The NSPCC has analysed police force data and has found that comparable statistics show that child cruelty rates have doubled in the last five years. Between 2017/ 2018 there were 14,263 cases reported and between 2022/2023 there were 29,422 cases reported.

These offences involve adults neglecting, mistreating or assaulting children. The NSPCC asks the government for a total reform of children's social care. Their chief executive, Sir |Peter Wanless said: "These latest child cruelty figures are a stark wake-up call that our current system is struggling to prevent the horrifying abuse and neglect happening to some of the youngest and most vulnerable in our society." He goes on to say that the government has in fact promised to reform the system and to provide earlier support in order to stop families from reaching crisis point.

Well yes I expect they have. But as yet we see no signs whatsoever of this happening as the above pages bear witness.

****

*"Childhood should be carefree,
playing in the sun; not living
a nightmare in the darkness
of the soul."*

Dave Pelzer. A Child Called "It"

******

CHILDREN AND HEALTH

In 2020, the Royal College of Paediatrics and Child Health (RCPCH) published 'State of Child Health 2020.' It showed a bleak picture; worsening health outcomes across indicators including obesity, mental health and child poverty, and widening inequalities in these health outcomes.

They said that there is no time to be lost; "Government must tackle the state of child health across the UK head-on, taking a cross-government approach and ensuring all Government departments work together towards the same aim of ensuring all children get the best start in life. If the Government wants to truly level up the country, they should use child health outcomes as their measure of progress. In doing so, children's life changes will improve, poverty will be reduced and so too will the economic prosperity of the country in the future."

The report made a number of evidence-based policy recommendations in addition to data analysis, which reflected three key priorities the Government must adopt in order to improve child health outcomes across the UK:

- Reduce health inequalities.
- Prioritise public health, prevention and early intervention.
- Build and strengthen local, cross-sector services to reflect local need.

"What unites these priorities is the need to consider the impacts of all policies on child health outcomes, not just those policies that fall under the remit of the Department of Health and Social Care."

Indeed in all of the chapters in this book the health of children is impacted.

As they go on to say, "There are few areas of policy that do not – whether intentionally or not – affect child health outcomes. Data consistently show that poverty and inequality impact a child's whole life, affecting their educational attainment, housing and social environment across the life course, in turn impacting their health outcomes and life chances."

'State of Child Health' also made a number of recommendations to paediatricians to improve their practice. "But," they say "the reality is that much of child health outcomes are socially determined. Our members want, need and deserve for Government to step up and play their part."

CHILD OBESITY

This is an on-going problem which this government seems to have no desire to fix.

Health campaigners are disappointed that there is no plan to curb the sale of junk food or any conversation at all about heavily processed food.

The government has already delayed its planned ban on two-for-one junk food deals – a key anti-obesity measure – until 2025. These are items which have high salt, fat and sugar content. There is concern that this measure could be dropped completely and the fact that it was not mentioned in Sunak's speech to the party conference would certainly suggest that it is not a priority.

This, at a time when data is showing that there is an increase in the proportion of 4-5 year olds recorded as overweight or obese in

England. As the report says, **"Nearly one-third of England's most deprived boys will be obese in 2030 if the Government's Childhood Obesity Plan is not implemented."**

But there are other trends which they report which are equally concerning.

They say that "England has poorer health outcomes than the average across the EU15+ (the 15 EU countries in 2004 plus Canada, Australia and Norway) in most areas studied, and the rate of improvement in England for many outcomes is lower than across the EU15+. This means that unless current trends improve, England is likely to fall further behind other wealthy countries over the next decade. The marked inequalities observed in most key outcomes are likely to widen over the next decade as problems in areas such as **infant mortality and obesity are worsening more quickly amongst the most deprived section of the population.**"

Then in late December, less than three weeks into her new role as health secretary, we near that Victoria Atkins has said that she is very unlikely to take any significant action and that all that people needed was good nutritional and dietary advice. Health campaigners are furious. The obesity crisis, they say, will never be resolved by just giving ideas as to what to eat and what to avoid.

A new report commissioned by the government actually interviewed over 100 people and in actual fact they all knew what constitutes a healthy diet but are trapped into making poor decisions and buying unhealthy food because of the promotion of cheap junk food and the comparatively higher costs of healthier options.

Tam Fry, chair of the 'National, Obesity Forum' but who, for some reason was not involved with this report, said that unless action is taken to curb the attraction and availability of ultra-processed food and foods high in fat, sugar and salt "then their most serious by-product –namely obesity—will continue to rise."

I say always follow the money. Our new health secretary, remember her name, Victoria Atkins, is married to Paul Kenwood who just happens to be CEO of ABF Sugar. ABF sugar is one of the world's leading sugar businesses which operates 27 plants in 10 countries and have 32,000 employees. They have the capacity to produce some 4.5 million tonnes of sugar annually.

She absolutely denies any conflict of interest.

****

SMOKING AND VAPING

Mr. Sunak has just announced that he is to set up a plan to make it illegal to sell young people cigarettes. He wants to ban smoking. Well that is a fine objective but am not sure how that can be enforced. There is a huge backlash about this. People are saying that it will all just go onto the black market. The way he is going to do it is to ban it year by year rather than an all-out ban. So you will get a situation where-by, for example a 23 year old will not be able to smoke but a 24 year old will be.

Hmm can't see that one working out. Smoking is already pretty much socially unacceptable and I have always thought that a school trip to a cancer ward would do it.

What about vaping then? I have just read this appalling story reported by the BBC.

Sarah Griffin is 12 years old. She suffered from asthma and was a heavy vaper when she was rushed to hospital with breathing problems a month ago. Sarah had started vaping when she was just nine. Her mum Mary told the BBC she feared she was going to lose her daughter.

She suffered a lung collapse and spent four days in an induced coma. Her mother has told the BBC that children should never start vaping.

Recent figures suggest that one in five children aged 15-17 have now tried vaping - three times as many as in 2020.

Vaping among younger children is also rising, with nearly one in ten 11- to 15-year-olds using them, according to a 2021 survey.

Sarah Woolnough, from charity 'Asthma + Lung UK,' said she wanted to see restrictions on the marketing of vapes so that they did not target children.

"Disposable vapes at their current pocket money prices, with cartoons and bubble-gum flavour options, are far too attractive and easy for children to access," she said.

Professor Chris Whitty, England's chief medical officer, said marketing vapes or e-cigarettes to children was "utterly unacceptable".

But it is actually illegal to sell vapes to anyone under 18 so why are the manufacturers allowed to actively target children?

Trading standards in England and Wales say the market is being flooded by unsafe, disposable vapes purposely aimed at children.

Doctors warned that the colourful, sweet-flavoured devices are growing in popularity among teens and more should be done to protect them from illegal and unregulated products containing high levels of nicotine.

And Helen Donegan, senior trading standards officer with Leicestershire County Council, said that large numbers of vapes which are not designed for the UK market, are being smuggled into the country. "There's no way of knowing what's in them," she said and 8,000 illegal vapes had been found at one premises alone.

Some look very similar to big-name vape brands, but are fake - others contain illegal amounts of nicotine and e-liquid. Instead of containing around 600 puffs, which is what UK regulations allow, disposable vape devices containing up to 10,000 puffs are being sold in the UK.

Dominic, 17, from Newcastle, has been vaping since he was 15, after switching from smoking when his friends started using vapes: "Most of my friends vape or smoke - about 90%." he said.

Secondary school teachers are noticing the problem too. A recent survey of 3,000 found half have caught a pupil vaping in school in the last year, and one in five teachers said they'd caught a pupil as young as 11 with a vape.

The charity 'ASH' says more should be done to prevent the products being promoted widely on platforms like TikTok.

"The flood of glamorous promotion of vaping on social media is completely inappropriate and social media platforms should take responsibility and turn off the tap," said chief executive Deborah Arnott.

The UK Vaping Industry Association wants the government "to greatly increase fines to £10,000" every time a shop is caught selling vapes to children.

It is also calling for outlets selling vape products to be licensed, and the fee used to fund further trading enforcement efforts by Trading Standards.

So what is the government going to do about it?

Well they have just announced a UK-wide consultation on its proposals to crack down on vaping among young people. How long will that take for goodness sake? We all know what needs to be done so why don't they?

The proposals include:

- Restricting the flavours and descriptions of vapes so they are no longer targeted at children.

- Keeping vapes out of sight of children in shops.

- Regulating vape packaging so they are not targeted at children.

- Exploring whether increasing the price of vapes will reduce the number of young people using them.

- Considering restricting the sale of disposable vapes, which ministers say are clearly linked to the rise in vaping in children and are incredibly harmful to the environment.

Pathetic is what I say to that. Read those words......"exploring, considering". Does that sound like a dynamic response to a problem that is putting young children into hospital with collapsed lungs and near fatality? No it does not. It sounds like a government that is weak and useless, has lost its momentum and is just marking time.

And yes indeed for we hear in the King's speech at the State Opening of Parliament (7th November 2023) the plans to prevent young people from smoking or vaping were announced. But there is no sense of urgency. It will take ages for this bill to become law.

For we read a report on the 6th November which said that there has been a big rise in hospital admissions linked to vaping for **children under the age of ten** since the start of last year. Dr Mike McKean, vice president for policy at the Royal College of Paediatrics and Child Health, said he was worried about the impact of "wholly avoidable hospitalisations" due to vaping on health services before the busy winter period.

Nicholas Hopkinson, professor of respiratory medicine and chairman of 'ASH', said: "Although this isn't on the scale of passive smoking, which causes around 5,000 children to be admitted to hospital every year in this country, any hospital admission is a concern.

"The simple message is that growing lungs need to breathe clean air. In young people, vaping can cause irritation to the airways in the lung and aggravate asthma. We know what worked to bring down smoking rates in early teens. Vaping needs the same approach, taking steps to reduce the affordability, accessibility and appeal of vapes to keep them out of the hands of children."

Professor Hopkison said it was "unfortunate" that the government had voted down amendments to the health and social care bill two years ago which would have given it powers to regulate the marketing of e-cigarettes to children, and prevent the distribution of free samples to under-18s.

Well I would not call it "unfortunate". I would call it once again, criminal negligence. A complete disregard for the lives of our children.

****

And then today (15th December 2023) the headlines are saying **"Pro-vaping campaign funded by Big Tobacco."** Investigative journalists at the *Times* have found that tobacco companies have funded scientific papers on vaping that play down the risks to children of vaping. Well of course. It is all profit to them and yes we must always follow the money.

Reuters says that: "Big tobacco firms shifting to new nicotine products, including Philip Morris International and British American Tobacco, have the most to lose if tobacco alternatives face the same rules as cigarettes."

And this is what I wrote in '**Britain Betrayed'** on page 182 in the part about the Institute of Economic Affairs (IEA) which is a right wing think tank.

"Many of you will be shocked to find that EU bureaucrats will be replaced by American executives in the tobacco industry, the (cane) sugar industry, the agrochemical industry, animal husbandry and

of course the fossil fuel industry via policies that, just as with the Brexit referendum, were discussed in secret outside parliament and cabinet.

Control was certainly taken back, all the way back to the neocon paymasters who've funded the greatest scam in British political history and they're nowhere near finished yet.

And I have not finished yet either.

"A BMJ (British Medical Journal) investigation includes infographic charts and diagrams which plot the IEA's financial links to 32 Tory MPs, and argues that the person most closely and publicly associated ideologically with the IEA is one-time Tory leadership candidate............. drum roll............. Dominic Raab. The BMA study also states that although he 'does not have direct links with the IEA', (former) health secretary (and another failed Tory leadership candidate) 'Matt Hancock has in recent years received funding [totalling £32,000] from Neil Record, who became chair of the IEA in 2015.' Well does any of this surprise you? It certainly explains a lot."

Our children need much more vigorous help from a concerned government.

****

The 'State of Child Health Report' goes on to say:

MORTALITY

"If infant mortality begins to decline again at its previous rate, rates will be 80% higher than the EU15+ in 2030. If UK mortality continues the current 'stall' then it will be 140% higher in 2030.

England and Wales had notably high mortality for one to 19-year-olds for chronic respiratory conditions (e.g. asthma) and epilepsy (2001-

2015) - mortality in both conditions is likely to remain substantially higher than the EU15+ average if current trends continue."

MENTAL HEALTH

"Reported mental health problems in England are set to increase by 63% in 2030 if recent trends continue.

ACCIDENT AND EMERGENCY ATTENDANCES

A&E attendances among children and young people are set to increase by 50% in 2030.

This report's overarching recommendation calls for "NHS England to develop a Children and Young People's Health Strategy for England, to be delivered by a funded transformation programme led by a dedicated programme board. The term 'health' encompasses physical health, mental health and wellbeing. This strategy should set out a governance and accountability framework for the commissioning, implementation and delivery of interventions to improve CYP health outcomes"

And then we see that the government appears to have taken notice of this report as the Health and Care Act 2022, was given Royal Assent on the 28th April 2022. This will apparently fundamentally change the way services are planned and delivered by the NHS, local authorities, and other key agencies

The most significant change relates to the expectations of the **42 Integrated Care Boards** (ICBs) that are replacing Clinical Commissioning Groups across the country from 1 July. Following a powerful intervention by members of the House of Lord, ICBs will now be required by the Act to set out the steps it will take to address the needs of children and young people under the age of 25 in their five-year forward plans. Children and young people are one of only two groups singled out by the primary legislation in this way.

So this is really encouraging.

But then I see a report by the 'King's Fund' written in **May 2022**. They say that "Most importantly this relies on people in systems and places continuing to learn how to work together, and that will need support, endurance and commitment long after the ink is dry on this Health and Care Act."

Indeed so. They also say that "you cannot run a health and care service without a work force and the evidence shows that years of poor planning have left deep shortages that leave the government struggling to deliver across the breadth of its health and care ambitions."

How often do we need to state that?

****

And here we are in 2023 so how is it all going?

Well of course the work force is still the main problem. In England, there were over **40 thousand vacancies** within the NHS nursing workforce in the first quarter of 2023 and thousands of doctors are planning to leave the NHS and go abroad to work due to the high levels of stress and the increasing work demands and the lack of any help or support or understanding from this government.

A 10-country survey has found that family GPs in the UK have some of the highest stress levels and lowest job satisfaction among the 10 countries and more than a third of GPs plan to quit their job in the next five years.

We still have strike after strike after strike with consultants on strike at the moment, October 2023. They have said they will call off the strikes immediately if the health secretary will get around a negotiating table and if he will call in ACAS. The then health secretary Steve Barclay, supported by the prime minister, refused to do this. He sat on his hands, blocked his ears and did nothing.

Meanwhile the waiting lists, already at an all-time high, continues to spiral out of control and children get the short straw.

On the 11th of May 2023 it was reported by the 'Patient Safety Learning –the Hub', that hospitals are failing to tackle spiralling children's surgery waiting lists as the backlog hits more than 400,000 for the first time. Leaked documents show children's waiting lists for both inpatient and outpatient care are "increasing at double the rate of adults" and, despite efforts, services have failed to catch up after they were paused during the pandemic.

Young people have been purposely 'deprioritised' on NHS waiting lists in order to cut the adult waiting lists. An article in the *Independent* on February 19th 2023 by their health correspondent Rebecca Thomas states that "the latest NHS data for December lays bare the parlous state of paediatric medicine, with NHS leaders and doctors warning that adult care is being prioritised over children's."

This will obviously worsen inequalities between adult and children's care and could affect children's future quality of life. Children will often need surgery at a very specific time in their lives in order for it to have the greatest long-term benefit so this is extremely worrying.

****

MALNUTRITION

The other issue that I find appalling is the fact that British five-year-olds are up to 7cm shorter than children of the same age in Europe. **In 2020, an Imperial College London team behind a study into the height of children up to the age of 19 warned that nutrition- and especially a lack of quality food - could be stunting the growth of children in the UK.** The data is taken from national measurement programmes, collated by the 'Non-Communicable Diseases Risk Factor Collaboration,' a global network of health scientists.

Professor Tim Cole, an expert in child growth rates at the Great Ormond Street Institute of Child Health, University College London, who was not involved in the most recent study, told *The Times* newspaper that wider data on the height of 19-year-olds suggested that growing up in the 2010s "which happens to coincide with the period of austerity . . . tells me that austerity has clobbered the height of children in the UK".

He said height was an extremely sensitive indicator of general living conditions, with factors including illness and infection, stress, poverty and sleep quality all "piled up in there" alongside the quality and quantity of diets.

"**It's quite clear we are falling behind, relative to Europe**," he added. "But it's telling that at age five, we are looking further behind than we are at age 19, which suggests to me that the last 14 years from age five to 19 has been particularly rough for UK children."

I say to the government have you read this report? I shout it at the top of my voice I am so angry, but no-one is listening.

Introducing free school meals as the Mayor of London, Sadiq Khan has just done this September, would help straight away.

More than 4 million children are living in poverty with 1 million being under 4 years old and yes, doctors are seeing children with severe malnutrition, and the return of rickets and scurvy in children due to the rise in the cost of living. They are pale and thin and have iron, folate and vitamin D deficiency.

Dayna Brackley is a senior food policy consultant at Bremner & Co, an organisation working to improve child health and nutrition. She is leading a review of early years' nutrition in the UK. She is also an MSc student at the Centre for Food Policy.

She writes in the *Independent* that, "In 2023 in the UK, the sixth wealthiest nation in the world (measured by GDP), the health outcomes of our children are dire. The statistics paint a devastating picture: 23.4 % of 11- to 12-year-olds are living with obesity (the prevalence is twice as high for those living in deprived areas), close to a quarter of 5-year-olds have dental decay and children who have been raised in the age of austerity are shorter than their European counterparts. Shorter, bigger and in poorer health. How did we get here?"

She rails against the government abandoning yet again the buy-one-get-one-free offers in supermarkets.

She emphasises the two main factors which, as we have seen are poverty and a poor diet, and says that we are doomed to fail because a healthy diet is just not affordable for many people. A recent report by the' Food Foundation' showed how the poorest fifth of the population would need to spend half of their disposable income to meet the government's diet recommendations.

The government's recommendations for our diet are simply not achievable for people living through a cost of living crisis.

****

CLIMATE CHANGE

Then there is the net zero policy on the climate crisis which is being kicked further and further down the road by Rishi Sunak. As I write this on October 23rd 2023, , the UK is reeling from a tremendous storm which has led to huge amounts of flooding, homes being evacuated and people dying.

I read a report in the *Guardian* by their Health Editor Andrew Gregory who quotes Dr. Camilla Kingdon as saying that "The climate crisis poses an "existential risk" to the health and wellbeing of all children and action to tackle it is needed immediately." She is the president of the Royal College of Paediatrics and Child Health (RCPCH) and Britain's most senior paediatrician and she attacked what she described as the rolling back of net zero policies by Rishi Sunak and said the country's most vulnerable children would be left bearing the greatest burden as a result.

"Every adolescent was at grave risk from the physical and mental effects of the climate crisis. Healthcare professionals were already seeing its impact first-hand," she added.

The report goes on to say that multiple studies have found rising temperatures around the world as a result of the climate crisis are having a devastating effect on foetuses, babies and children.

Scientists have determined that the climate emergency is causing – among other adverse outcomes – an increased risk of premature birth and hospitalisation of young children as well as weight gain in babies. Research shows pollution can stunt children's lung growth, cause asthma and affect blood pressure, cognitive abilities and mental health.

"Climate change is no longer tomorrow's problem, it's today's," Dr. Kingdon said. "Healthcare professionals across the UK are already seeing its impact first-hand."

In the UK, air pollution was the largest environmental risk to public health, she added. "Children breathe faster, so they inhale more airborne toxins in proportion to their weight than adults exposed to the same amount of air pollution. As such, they are especially vulnerable to air pollution, which can lead to asthma in childhood, and lifelong health issues."

She also talks about the mental health effects of climate change on children and says that "The mental health effects of climate change on children are significant and may be long lasting. Children exhibit high levels of concern over climate change and the mental health consequences, including post-traumatic stress disorder, depression, anxiety, phobias, sleep disorders, attachment disorders and substance abuse, can lead to problems with learning, behaviour, and academic performance."

And of course those on lower incomes have less choice in where they live, and the climate crisis is leading to more damp and cold properties as a result of increases in winter precipitation in the UK. For low-income households, homes may be too expensive to heat to an adequate temperature, increasing their exposure to cold and mould.

Dr. Kingdon said: "Every child is at grave risk of the effects of our changing climate, but none more so than children in lower-income families. These children are facing an increased mortality risk from extreme weather events, exacerbated respiratory conditions from dirty air and even increased rates of cancer, diabetes and obesity. It is wholly unjust that these vulnerable children should bear the greatest burden in terms of climate change, especially in the context of a government that is rolling back on its net zero policies."

The RCPCH wants Sunak to appoint a cabinet minister for children and to prioritise child health in policymaking on the climate crisis.

"We cannot continue like this as a country, with our heads in the sand," Dr. Kingdon said. "There is no such thing as the 'right time' economically to tackle climate change, and indeed the cost of not reaching net zero is far greater. We must act now and with our children in mind. As an organisation, we continue to call on political leaders to take action on poverty and health inequalities while also emphasising the unequal impact of climate change."

This is a dreadful criticism of an incompetent and vacuous government. And do we think that this government is listening? Of course not. They have just lost two local by-elections to huge unprecedented swings to Labour and they are just concerned in covering their own backs.

The welfare of our children is never on their agenda.

****

DENTAL CARE

And on Wednesday 19th July 2023 we hear that **about 27,000 children were on waiting lists for specialist dental care, assessments or procedures in January,** according to the figures obtained by the Liberal Democrats from the NHS Business Services Authority.

The figures cover NHS Community Dental Services. These are supposed to provide treatments to patients that require specialist dental care due to their specific needs.

These include children with special needs, children with physical or learning disabilities, children living in foster homes, children who are homeless, and children who are on "at risk" registers.

But the figures also includes children not in these categories whose untreated tooth decay has become so severe that they now require specific treatment for complex dental problems.

Daisy Cooper, the Liberal Democrat health spokesperson said "It is heartbreaking to think that some children are being left waiting in pain for months or even years for the specialised dental care they need. Every child deserves access to the dental care they need, regardless of where they live."

Over and over again we see dither and delay by a government who thinks it is more economical to put things off in the hope that it will all get better.

****

MATERNITY CARE

I now need to turn to our maternity services to find out how we welcome our children into the world and how we manage healthy outcomes for them all.

Shamefully it is not looking good as I am sure many of you will remember the inquiry into the maternity services at the Shrewsbury and Telford trust which was led by Donna Ockenden. This uncovered serious failings which saw 300 babies left dead or brain damaged by inadequate NHS care.

Other inquiries have laid bare more serious failures that have led to more mothers and babies being harmed and dying because of poor care provided by maternity services at the Morecambe Bay and East Kent NHS hospital trusts.

Now another one, into maternity care at the Nottingham hospital trust, once again being led by the midwifery expert Donna Ockenden, is also under way. It is expected to report next year (2024).

I think it is important to understand exactly what we are talking about so I quote a tiny part of the Ockenden report on the Shrewsbury and Telford Hospital Trust here.

"**Patterns of repeated poor care**.

Through the review of 1,486 family cases, the review team has been able to identify thematic patterns in the quality of care and investigation procedures carried out by the Trust, and identify where opportunities for learning and improving quality of care have been missed.

For example, in the nine months preceding the avoidable death of Kate Stanton-Davies in March 2009, the review team has identified two further incidents of baby deaths which occurred under similar circumstances.

"In May 2008 Baby Joshua was born in poor condition at Ludlow midwifery-led unit, and was transferred by air ambulance to the Royal Shrewsbury Hospital Neonatal Unit. Joshua's mother was considered to have a low risk pregnancy, and even after she reported episodes of severe uterine tenderness and tightening at 31 weeks this risk profile was not changed.

She reported reduced baby movements the day before her labour at 37+5 weeks gestation, but on her admission the baby's heart rate was not monitored appropriately. Joshua was delivered with no signs of life and died at six days old, when care was withdrawn.

"In January 2009 Baby Thomas was born following his mother's long, slow labour stretching over more than a day. His mother, who had given birth to a large baby during a previous pregnancy, had been treated as a low risk case throughout this pregnancy, and no check for gestational diabetes was conducted.

She had been due to give birth in a midwifery-led unit, but was admitted to the antenatal ward in the consultant-led unit. The review team found that despite abnormal heart rate readings, a high dose of oxytocin infusion was used, and she was infrequently monitored. In the hour before birth, examinations showed signs of obstructed labour and uterine rupture, as well as difficulties establishing the baby's heart rate, but despite this a vaginal delivery was attempted before an emergency caesarean was conducted. Thomas briefly had a heartbeat but at 34 minutes of age resuscitation was stopped.

"Then on 1 March 2009 Rhiannon Davies gave birth to Kate Stanton-Davies at the Ludlow midwifery-led unit, despite reporting a reduction in her baby's movements in the two weeks before the birth. There was a lack of appropriate heart rate monitoring during labour and missed opportunities to manage Kate's health as she was born severely anemic.

Kate suffered a cardiopulmonary collapse at 90 minutes of life and was transferred by air ambulance to a tertiary neonatal unit, where she died shortly after arrival at six hours of age.

"The review team found evidence of poor investigation into all three of these cases which took place within less than a year of each other, as well as a lack of transparency and dialogue with families. This resulted in missed opportunities for learning, and a lost opportunity to prevent further baby deaths from occurring at the

Trust. Unfortunately these three cases were not isolated incidents and throughout this review we have found repeated errors in care, which led to injury to either mothers or their babies. During our work we have considered all aspects of clinical care in maternity services including antenatal, intrapartum, postnatal, obstetric anaesthesia and neonatal care.

Most of the neonatal deaths occurred in the first 7 days of life. Nearly a third of all incidents reviewed (27.9 per cent) were identified to have significant or major concerns in the maternity care provided which might or would have resulted in a different outcome".

The report says that, "At the time of concluding this review, in total 19 maternal deaths were noted by the review team. Three of these occurred prior to the core review period (before 2000) and one death in 2015 occurred after the mother was transferred in labour to another trust. This woman's pregnancy care was reviewed by the team as the majority of the pregnancy care occurred at the Shrewsbury and Telford Trust's maternity services, but her death was not.

"Of the 16 cases that occurred within the core review period, there were eight direct, and seven indirect maternal deaths, plus one accidental death resulting from a road accident, which was not investigated further by the review team.

Although statistical analysis of the maternal deaths is limited due to the small numbers, the review team noted the relatively high number of direct maternal deaths at the Trust. This is in contrast to the overall national trend, where direct deaths have been declining since 2004. This may be an indication that the care for pregnancy related conditions such as pre-eclampsia sepsis and major obstetric haemorrhage needs to be further improved locally.

"The review team noted that several families felt their questions surrounding the maternal death had not been addressed by the Trust. Bereavement support after the event was also described by families as inconsistent."

This is a long and detailed report but the above is just a flavour of the findings and how distressing it has been.

In early April 2022 a group of 100 families affected by the alleged failings in maternity care at Nottingham University Hospitals NHS Trust, wrote a letter to the former Health Secretary Sajid Javid, voicing concerns about its performance with families.

The fact that Donna Ockenden has been asked to lead another inquiry so soon is absolutely heart-breaking.

****

Then we read further reports.

The BBC analysed the 'Care Quality Commission' safety ratings, published in September 2022, for 137 maternity units in England and found:

- Nine were given the lowest possible rating of inadequate for safety, meaning urgent action is required.

- 66 required improvement to reduce risk to mothers and babies, and ensure legal requirements on safety are met

- 62 had a good rating for safety

- None were given the top rating of outstanding that would mean a comprehensive safety system was in place,

- The figures are slightly worse than a few years ago, despite several attempts to transform maternity care.

The regulator says the pace of improvement has been disappointing.

I say it has been criminally negligent.

******

Rob Behrens, the **NHS ombudsman** for England voiced alarm that, although efforts have been made to improve the care mothers and their children receive, progress is too slow – and that means patients remain in danger.

His report says that: "We recognise that people working in maternity services want to provide high-quality care. Culture, systems and processes can get in the way of achieving that goal. But improvements are not happening quickly enough, and we have not seen sustainable change. We must do more to make services safer for everyone."

Mothers and babies are being put at risk because maternity services are still providing unsafe care, despite a series of scandals that have cost lives, the NHS ombudsman has warned.

More tragedies will occur unless the health service takes decisive action to put an end to repeated and deeply ingrained problems which lead to "the same mistakes over and over again", he said.

"The fact that we are seeing the same mistakes over and over again shows that lessons are not being learned. This is unacceptable. There needs to be significant improvements and change."

****

But the **Care Quality commission's** most recent annual report into maternity services in England in January this year **(2023)** said that **the quality of care had deteriorated in recent years.** It found that fewer mothers reported positively about their experience of maternity care, with a notable decline in the number able to get help from staff when they needed it, compared to five years ago. They were unable to get the help they needed at every stage of their care. They were not able to get advice about how to feed their baby during the evening, overnight and at weekends. They also felt that any concerns they raised during their labour or birth were not taken seriously.

In other words, yet again women's voices go unheard and the care is not improving.

****

But here is a report by' Save the Children'. It is their annual report published in 2018 and they noted that Japan, Iceland and Singapore "are the three safest countries in which to be born". High standards of living and guaranteed public access to a first rate public health system are among the keys to low levels of infant mortality. The report goes on to say that: "Countries such as Japan, Iceland and Singapore have strong, well-resourced health systems, ample numbers of highly skilled health workers, a well-developed infrastructure, readily available clean water and high standards of sanitation and hygiene in health facilities.

Public health education, combined with very high standards of medical care, guaranteed universal access to quality health care at all ages, and general standards of nutrition, education and environmental safety are also high. It is likely that all these factors contribute to very low new-born mortality rates."

Well that sounds amazing. My heart lifts when I read something like that. They all seem to be achievable goals in a first world country. And Finland too is a country which looks after its newborns.

I remember reading a devastating letter in the *Times* from Dr. Peter Green who was chairman of the 'National Network of Designated Healthcare Professionals for Children'. He wrote that, "if all the infants born in the UK in 2017 had been born in Finland as **many as 1,500 more would have survived.**" He said that "when assessed over the past decade, the statistics indicate well over 10,000 excess UK infant deaths in that time."

We just need a bit of time to absorb those details.

****

Then on the 5th April 2023 The RCM's Public Affairs Advisor, Stuart Bonar, explains how the midwife shortage in England is getting bigger, rather than smaller.

He says that "The NHS in England is short of 2,500 midwives. We can say that with confidence because it is not a figure plucked from thin air. This figure is the product of detailed analysis, looking at how many births are taking place, how many births are taking place in consultant-led units as opposed to midwife-led units or at home, how many midwives are in post, the need for specialist midwife roles, and other factors too. It is a constantly changing situation, and for that reason the RCM regularly looks at how it calculates how many midwives the NHS needs and refreshes its calculation."

It paints a stark picture of chronic workforce shortages and challenges with maternity services often only functioning safely because of staff working long and additional hours, often unpaid.

The Royal College of Midwives says it also shows a service haemorrhaging midwives at an alarming rate. "The loss of experienced midwives is impacting on the ability to support and train student midwives on their placements in the NHS. They are leaving because they cannot deliver the quality of care they so desperately want, because of their falling pay, and because they are exhausted, fragile and burnt-out."

But nothing seems to improve. Does no-one ever read these reports?

Dr. Suzanne Tyler of the Royal College of Midwives said: "Report after report has made a direct connection between staffing levels and safety, yet the midwife shortage is worsening. Midwives are desperately trying to plug the gaps – in England alone we estimate that midwives work around 100,000 extra unpaid hours a week to keep maternity services safe. This is clearly unsustainable and now is the time for the chancellor to put his hand in the Treasury pocket and give maternity services the funding that is so desperately needed."

She said "Our worst fears about where we saw maternity services heading are becoming a reality and the fault lies squarely at the door of successive Conservative Governments. Chronic understaffing is hitting the morale of midwives and maternity support workers (MSW) and the safety of care. They are leaving in droves and the Government must plug this worrying leak as a matter of real urgency. Improving pay, more investment and increasing the workforce are crucial to building back our shattered maternity services. The Government must do that now and it can start with giving maternity staff the inflation busting pay award they deserve."

Well we won't hold our breath.

****

We won't hold our breath because we see this from the Department of Health.

A spokesperson said: "The NHS is already one of the safest places to give birth in the world, but there is more to do. We've taken steps to improve the quality of care, with £165m of extra investment a year. This includes funding to increase the number of midwifery posts available.

"NHS England has also published its three-year delivery plan for maternity and neonatal services, which will make maternity and neonatal care safer and more personalised for all women, babies and families."

This is the plan put out on the 4th April 2023.

"This plan sets out how the NHS will make maternity and neonatal care safer, more personalised, and more equitable for women, babies, and families. There was clear agreement on what the plan's focus should be, so for the next three years, services are asked to concentrate on four themes:

- Listening to and working with women and families, with compassion
- Growing, retaining, and supporting our workforce
- Developing and sustaining a culture of safety, learning, and support
- Standards and structures that underpin safer, more personalised, and more equitable care.

Delivering this plan will continue to require the dedication of everyone working in NHS maternity and neonatal services in England who are working tirelessly to support women and families and improve care."

I honestly do not know how they have the gall to say this. They do not need to increase the number of midwifery posts -- just filling the existing vacancies would be a good start. And to say they require the dedication of everyone working in maternity services is frankly insulting. They are on their knees and working all hours for very little pay and are burnt out.

The latest Ockenden report should be out next year so we will see whether any lessons have been learnt.

But just today (**October 13th 2023**) I read this report. An independent review into maternity deaths says that 241 women died during pregnancy and within six weeks of giving birth between 2019 and 2021. It includes 17 women who bled to death, 23 who died of sepsis and 33 who died of Covid. A further 331 died in the 12 months after giving birth with suicide being the leading cause.

The report says that half of these deaths were potentially avoidable had the women received better care amid a deterioration in NHS maternity services. Maternal deaths have increased by 15 % since 2009 which means the government will probably miss its target of halving maternal mortality by 2025. This research was by MBRRACE-UK (Mothers and Babies: Reducing Risk through Audits and Confidential Enquiries across the UK) which is a collaboration of academics. They said that women in deprived areas were twice as likely to die than those in wealthy areas and black women were four times as likely to die as white women.

The report recommends speedier recognition of potentially fatal bleeding and greater mental health support for vulnerable women after giving birth. Well yes that would undoubtedly help.

And today (**31st October 2023**) I see that bereaved parents whose babies have died because of failures by the NHS are calling for a public inquiry into the poor maternity services. The 'Maternity Safety Alliance' has written to Steve Barclay to say that the inquiry must look at the "true scale of maternity care failings" and "tackle rotten culture, including women not being listened to, lack of care and respect and 'normal birth' ideology". They are a "group of bereaved parents, other family members, and maternity safety campaigners from across the country, brought together by our shared mission to ensure every mum and every baby receives safe and compassionate maternity care."

This inquiry is essential but should have happened years ago.

****

And also at the end of this month I see that The 'Care Quality Commission' has rated 65% of maternity services in England as either "inadequate" or "requires improvement" for the safety of care – up from 54% last year. "Services are beset by a host of problems, including serious staff shortages and internal tensions, which mean that too many mothers and their babies receive care that is not good enough," it said.

There is a "deteriorating picture in maternity services", said Kate Terroni, its interim deputy chief executive.

Well, all the above would certainly verify this and it is a horrifying picture of negligence, incompetence and under-funding.

And just today (**November 28th 2023**) we read about yet another case of negligence causing the preventable death of a new-born baby as a woman in labour was misdiagnosed **over the phone** in January this year. **She had a severe case of internal bleeding but was told by over-worked, and highly pressured mid-wives that it was probably a "panic attack".**

When, oh when will they listen to the women who know their own bodies best?

****

FORMULA MILK

But just before we leave the well-being of our babies I see this. A mother is in tears because she cannot afford baby milk formula for her baby and food banks are having to ration formula milk.

Baby banks are being forced to ration formula milk because of soaring demand caused by desperate parents struggling to afford the rising cost of the product in stores.

Data from 'First Steps Nutrition' showed average prices for baby formula rose by 22 % between March 2021 and April 2023, with the cost of feeding a 10-week-old baby as of August this year costing up to £89 per month.

One baby bank in Swindon told *Sky News* it is now having to ration families to just one tub of formula per week, while High Peak Baby Bank in Derbyshire said it has restricted families to three tubs a month.

Parents have called for more help from Westminster, with one saying ministers "are not listening".

How often do we accuse them of that?

One mother told *Sky News* at the Swindon baby bank that, even with her maternity pay combined with her partner's wage, they are still unable to afford baby essentials. "It is literally a milk crisis," she said. "It makes me feel so angry and irritated that parents are forced to feel ashamed that they can't afford milk for their babies. The government are not listening."

Another mother told the broadcaster: "Please help, help those mums, help those dads. Don't ask questions, just do. Don't sit there and judge and look and ponder just do it. It's as simple as that."

I saw a reporter questioning an MP and asking what his advice is to this distraught mother who was in tears as her food bank was rationing formula milk. His reply was that the government was determined to bring down inflation and that would result in bringing prices down and so that was the best way forward.

So to all desperate mothers please just explain to your 4 month old babies that they will have to wait for inflation to come down. And no that probably won't happen before tonight's feed I'm afraid so, my baby, you will just have to cry the whole night through.

The face of compassionate Conservatism.

****

DANGEROUS DRUG WHEN PREGNANT

On **October 23rd 2022** on page 67 in my book "**Britain Betrayed**" I wrote about a drug called **sodium valproate.** This is a drug used to treat epilepsy and bipolar disorder. However it must never be given to pregnant women as it causes disabilities and deformities in new born babies. NHS data shows that 286 pregnant women were prescribed this drug between April 2018 and March 2022 exposing many unborn babies to its damaging effects.

It is estimated that 20,000 children in the UK have been damaged since the 1970s.

I wrote about the fact that Jeremy Hunt, who was then chairman of the health committee, backed calls for compensation but campaigners had meetings cancelled and emails and phone calls not responded to due to inaction at the heart of government because of the ongoing changes of Prime Ministers. And there were still none of the legally required warnings on the packets of this drug,

In fact on September 2nd 2022 Hunt said: "It is incredibly concerning to know that women of child-bearing age can still be prescribed the epilepsy drug sodium valproate despite its known risks as a cause of birth defects or developmental delays. It has been two years since Baroness Cumberlege called for urgent action to prevent this happening. However, dozens of pregnant women were prescribed the drug last year while data published last month has shown that safety requirements were not being fully met.

We're calling on a Minister and senior health officials as well as campaigners to address our concerns."

Today is the 19th November 2023 and we are hearing that this drug is still being given to pregnant women. There has just been a report in the *Sunday Times* by Shan Lintern their health editor about it all but I see that in February this year the Pharmaceutical Journal was writing about it and reported Henrietta Hughes, the patient safety commissioner, as saying that it was "**a far bigger scandal than thalidomide**" and, since her appointment in **2022, she has continued to urge the government to "not kick this issue into the long grass".**

But the long grass is completely over-grown with all the lost policies of the Conservative government.

Dr. Hughes was appalled to hear that it was only **after** women became pregnant that they were told about the dangers of this drug. She also predicted that without a system to monitor drugs such as this one, other drug scandals could occur.

I say in my previous book that women, and especially those of child-bearing years are never listened to but.................. wait a minute......................... what is this I see?

Men taking the drug for epilepsy could also have problems.

The MHRA (Medicines and Healthcare products Regulatory Agency) highlighted that there are emerging risks to male sperm from valproate, as well as fertility issues though apparently that "can be reversed once the drug is stopped". These risks, it said, could affect 100,000 males taking sodium valproate.

Well there you go. I think we can expect immediate action now.

****

I discover another charity. It is called 'Together for Short Lives'. On their website they state that: "Together for Short Lives' purpose is to ensure that every seriously ill child, and their family, has high quality children's palliative and end of life care, when and where they need it. That's what drives us to do the work we do."

They go on to say that: "Through our family support team and helpline we provide families of seriously ill children with emotional, financial and practical support and advice. We champion and support palliative care professionals with training and resources. We work to influence policy making and Government to secure more investment in children's palliative care. And through working with our corporate partners we raise £millions to support local children's hospices directly. Our vision is that every family caring for a seriously ill child has access to the high-quality care and support they need, when and where they need it."

But this amazing charity has discovered, by using the freedom of information laws, that there is a damaging postcode lottery when it comes to funding children's hospice care. They found that a child in South Yorkshire had £28 spent on its services as opposed to a child in Norfolk who had £511 spent on each of them.

And 14% of the local bodies had no record at all of the amount they had spent. They also found that local NHS systems had a complete lack of records on the number of children who needed palliative care or who were using the services.

There are nearly 100,000 babies, children and young people in the UK who have health conditions which are life limiting or life-threatening.

Andy Fletcher, their chief executive, said "The variation in NHS funding for children who need hospice care is a real concern". He goes on to say that: "The government should urgently introduce long-term, fair and transparent funding to sustain crucial palliative and services for children and their families in hospitals, homes and hospices."

Legislation was introduced last year which created a duty for local NHS services to fund and plan palliative and end of life care. It would appear that nothing has been done.

In fact I discover that NHS England wrote to children's hospices in April to tell them that this year (2023/24) will be the final year of the NHSE Children's Hospice Grant – and that local integrated care boards (ICBs) would be responsible for providing all of their NHS funding in future.

I write about the introduction of these integrated health boards on page 74. They were legally established in July 2022. There are 42 in England and they consist of "local partnerships that bring health and care organisations together to develop shared plans and joined-up services. They are formed by NHS organisations and upper-tier local councils in each area and also include the voluntary sector, social care providers and other partners with a role in improving local health and wellbeing."

Well that is the blurb on the NHS England web site. However would it surprise you to hear that currently ICB funding is patchy and nowhere near the level that will sustain the crucial hospice services that children and families need. It is not enough and TFSL say the effect of this will be that:-

Nearly 38% of children's hospices would cut end of life care they provide. One would stop providing it altogether.

Nearly 79% would cut the respite or short breaks they provide and one would stop providing them altogether.

66% would cut the hospice at home services they provide. One would stop providing them altogether.

Their voices need to be heard by everyone involved.

This is yet more unbelievable negligence of our most vulnerable children and this charity is doing amazing work in order to improve the lives of seriously ill young people.

******

MENTAL HEALTH ISSUES

According to NHS figures in a report on the mental health of children and young people in England, overall **one in five older teenage girls have an eating disorder**. Rates have risen since 2017 in both young women and to a lower extent in young men and Tom Quinn director of external affairs at the eating disorder charity 'Beat' says "urgent action is needed."

The survey found unsurprisingly that there were higher rates of mental health problems in families who were struggling financially and who were, for example, unable to pay for their children to take part in activities outside school.

But schools too needed more investment to be able to equip young people with the skills they need to transition from school to early adult life. Of course lockdowns played a part but many children have been failed by the system and "allowed to fall through the cracks and become even more unwell."

The survey was conducted by the 'Office for National Statistics, the National Centre for Social Research', and the universities of Cambridge and Exeter.

Too often, girls especially, are praised for their looks and so worry about growing up and transitioning into adulthood and develop anxiety issues. Research suggests that this should be seen as a mental health problem rather than a problem about food.

******

So the health of our children seems to be being compromised on so many levels. The NHS is working against all odds to look after our children and can still perform miracles but they are on their knees and forecasting a winter which will be worse than ever. Then there are still so many plans they need to be concentrating on but obviously do not have the work-force to be able to do so. As I have reported we now have a new health secretary but the incompetence just goes on and on.

****

*"It is easier to build strong
children than to repair
broken men."*

Frederick Douglass, abolitionist and statesman

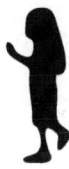

CHILDREN AND PRISON

Have you ever asked yourself the question "what happens to young children when their parents go to prison?"

No? Neither had I. I have been a member of the 'Howard League for Prison Reform' for nearly 40 years and I know all about the scandals of women in prison and children in Young Offender Institutes but I had never given a thought to children left on their own because their single parent was in jail.

But according to 'Keeping Children Safe in Education' which is the statutory guidance for schools and colleges from the Department of Education, 200,000 children have a parent in prison but the 'National Information Centre on Children of Offenders' estimates that the figure is closer to 310,000 and also say that 10,000 children visit public prisons every week.

But would it surprise you to know that there is no formal record kept of who these children might be and therefore we hear of many young children left to struggle at home on their own?

"This lack of robust research is a key barrier to offering such children the support they need," according to James Ottley, family and project operational manager at 'Children Heard And Seen' (CHAS) which is the wonderful name of an excellent charity which provides support to children and families impacted by parental imprisonment.

"There isn't the data, there isn't the funding and it seems like there isn't the interest," says Mr. Ottley, adding that this feels like purposeful avoidance by the government.

Yes I think we can all relate to that.

"By identifying how many children of prisoners there are, then you'd have to do something about it. By not identifying it, it's not a problem." He believes that children of prisoners should be eligible for the government's 'pupil premium' – a grant to improve educational outcomes for disadvantaged children, including those in the military. With the extra funding the premium provides, schools would have the capacity to offer individualised, expert support, such as educational psychologists and therapists.

Dr Shona Minson from the 'Centre for Criminology' at Oxford University agrees that suspended and deferred sentencing are both options that should be used more, and that short sentences should be abolished entirely, particularly for mothers. Some 70% of prison sentences handed to women are for less than 12 months, but spending just a few months in prison is enough for a mother to lose her home and often her children, she says. "The mother is in a catch-22 situation when released from prison as she is recorded as 'intentionally homeless', meaning she doesn't get housing priority, meaning she's placed in a single room in a hostel, and she's not eligible to have her children back. The impact on children, who often bounce from one care arrangement to another, is severe," she adds. "The sheer cruelty and negligence is beyond belief."

So many children have to deal with the shame, stigma, isolation and loneliness that this situation provokes. Some are bullied at school, others face violent attacks on their home. One story that particular resonated with me was that of a five-year-old boy who was the only one not invited to a classmate's birthday.

Often, understandably, parents fail to inform social services that there is a child at home after their arrests for fear of losing their child altogether.

But there are some shocking discoveries.

There was a 15-year-old boy, who had been alone for months – with no gas or electricity – after his mother had been jailed.

Another time, a victim support officer visited the home of a teenage girl, only to find she had been alone since her father's arrest.

A third time, a criminologist visiting a house for research purposes found just children living there.

Then there was Layla, who when she was eight – along with her six siblings – lived for several weeks without any parent or carer after her mother was arrested. "No one cared enough about who was going to look after us, we just got left," Layla, now 21, said. Her ten-year old sister was the eldest and "took on the whole clan". It was only when they took their malnourished six-month-old sister to the hospital that anyone realised their situation. "I received little to no support during the process of my mum being arrested and going to jail" she said. "This impacted me hugely and I still struggle with attachment issues, poor mental health and poor physical health."

This is obviously just the tip of the iceberg as so many children are completely abandoned.

And again, obviously, the ongoing harm is huge.

As 'CHAS' reports:-

65% of boys with a convicted parent go on to offend themselves.

25% of children with a parent in prison are at risk of mental health problems including depression, anxiety, eating and sleeping disorders.

So many suffer from bullying, truancy and failure to achieve in education.

And 69% of children with parents in prison do not visit the prison at all.

The prison population has risen by 80% in the last three decades and has grown substantially in the last few years, returning to levels not seen for over a decade. It is projected to rise by a further 7,400 by 2024.

And the average custodial sentence has increased by 57% since the Conservatives entered power in the coalition government in 2010.

Children's welfare is never considered.

Of course we hear this government going on about the 20,000 extra new prison places they are building but the reality is these plans have been put on hold due to lack of planning permission and will not be completed till at least 2030. And there are not enough prison staff at the moment.

Have they thought about where the extra staff will come from?

In fact just listen to this. They have been talking to Estonia and Norway about renting prison space as our prisons are now full.

Ahh, and what processes are being put in place for children to visit their parents there I wonder?

Of course as we keep saying mothers should not be incarcerated in prison and short-term sentences should be abolished.

And just two days ago on the 9th October (2023) Andrea Albutt the president of the Prison Governors Association used her valedictory conference address to berate politicians for reducing the Prison Service to "lunacy", prioritising an ever greater need for spaces over the health and safety of people living and working in jails.

She said that the likes of David Gauke and Rory Stewart, when justice secretary and prisons minister respectively, made the "brave decision" to end short-term sentences, but did not last in their posts. So this in fact never happened.

"The rightwing lurch by government has resulted in a populist rhetoric on prisons and we are now bust on prison places," she said. "While the government plans to build 20,000 new prison spaces, it cannot recruit enough staff for the current capacity and older jails are not fit for purpose."

Actually on top of everything else many of them are riddled with RAAC concrete.

****

In **September 2019** there was a report by a House of Commons Committee entitled "The Right to Family Life: children whose mothers are in prison."

This report states that although judges are required to consider primary caring responsibilities roughly 17,000 children each year are being harmed when their mothers are sent to prison. They say that "Children feel invisible in the sentencing process and in many cases they are indeed disregarded."

"Invisible". That one word describes the attitude of this government to all our children in every single chapter in this book.

In this case however the problem appears to be partly because the court does not have the correct information about whether the defendant has children and what the impact of a custodial sentence would be on them.

Their key recommendations to the government were:-

• that the Department for Education, working closely with the Ministry of Justice, must revise the framework for safeguarding and promoting the welfare of children so that much greater attention is paid to the needs of children and their families when mothers go to prison;

- that kinship carers who step in to care for children when their mothers go to prison should be entitled to financial and practical support;

- that mothers should, wherever possible and practicable, be placed in prisons close to their homes and non-means tested financial help should be made available to allow children to visit their mothers (or primary carers) in prison; and

- that contact should (other than in exceptional circumstances) be based on a child's right to respect for family life rather than premised on their mother's behaviour in prison.

Well that sounds reasonable to start off with, although I would prefer them to say that:-

- We recommend that all short-term prison sentences should be repealed.
- Pregnant woman should never be given a custodial sentence.

However they go on to say that: "We expect the Government to act swiftly in each of these areas in order to prevent another generation of children suffering the irreparable harm caused when mothers go to prison."

"Sending a mother to prison has a serious, detrimental impact on her children. This has been known for a long time. **In 1813 Elizabeth Fry visited Newgate Prison and protested at children being held in abysmal conditions alongside their imprisoned mothers.**"

Well no one can ever accuse, not just this government but successive governments since 1813, of being too hasty in their reform of prisons and the treatment of our children.

We then hear about the government's response in November 2019. Here is some of it presented to Parliament by the Lord Chancellor and Secretary of State for Justice.

I warn you it is very equivocal.

This is about the pre-sentencing reports.

"Given the range of factors that judges must already take into account in sentencing, the existing case-law and guidance already provided to the judiciary, **we do not believe that sentencers should be subject to a further explicit statutory obligation to consider the welfare of offenders' children when sentencing.** We are, however, prepared to ask the Criminal Procedure Rule Committee to consider making recommendations in light of the proposals made by the JCHR.

"However, we do agree with the committee's conclusion that it is vital that high quality pre-sentence reports (PSRs) are made available to sentencers by the National Probation Service to support sentencing decisions in line with these frameworks.

"**As the committee notes, the number of PSRs recorded as a percentage of sentences has steadily declined since 2012.** Currently, we are reviewing some cases where women were sentenced to custody without a report to see if we can identify any common themes.

"However, we acknowledge that the decline in the use of the pre-sentence reports may mean that opportunities are missed to inform sentencers where a defendant is a primary carer and of the impacts of custody on the child."

This is about child-care.

"Currently, the opportunity is available to make childcare arrangements or make contact with dependents or family members from court custody suites after sentencing. Whilst there are examples where this practice takes place, we acknowledge as per findings from Lord Farmer's 'Review for Women' that this may not always be the case, **as there is not yet a specific requirement for this to be supported.** We will be reviewing operational guidance across custody suites to ensure this process is formalised and consistent"

This is about problems with distances from the home.

"We acknowledge that distance from home can be a real challenge for the maintenance of these ties, and that this is particularly acute in the female estate. HMPPS is committed to ensuring that prisoners are accommodated as close as possible to their resettlement communities and families. This is not always possible due to a variety of factors including wider population pressures, or where individuals have specific sentence planning needs which can only be met at certain establishments."

And on visiting.

"All people in custody have a statutory entitlement to visits. Under the Prison Rules 1999 and Young Offender Institution Rules 2000 a convicted prisoner is entitled to receive a visit twice in every period of four weeks; un-convicted prisoners are allowed visits on at least three days a week, which includes weekends."

PREGNANT WOMEN

"This Government takes very seriously its responsibility for securing quality care for women prisoners who are pregnant, give birth or are caring for their new born babies whilst serving a custodial sentence. We will give careful consideration to any learning from the investigations into the infant death at Bronzefield."

"A perinatal pathway is currently being developed and applied across the entire estate, building on the excellent maternity service that HMP Low Newton has developed in conjunction with County Durham and Darlington NHS Foundation Trust. We are expecting full roll out across the women's estate from 2020 onward."

"These recommendations have been accepted by the Ministry of Justice and we are considering how these can best be taken forward."

Goodness. An "excellent maternity service"? Soon they will be saying it is safer to give birth in prison than in an NHS maternity ward.

So how quickly do we see change in the way this country treats women and children in prison?

Well in January 2022 Rona Epstein writes in the *Guardian:-*

"How many more babies must die before England stops jailing pregnant women?"

She writes that "sending pregnant women to prison is unnecessary. Multiple countries including Russia, Brazil, Mexico and Columbia already have laws to prevent pregnant women going to prison. It is time for the UK to follow their example."

There are many alternatives to prison and these need to be looked at very carefully. These women need support not incarceration and the probation service should help them to access this. It could turn their lives around in the way that prison never can.

Then in March 2023 the 'Nuffield Trust' writes that "The Sentencing Council is due to review whether there is a need for new guidance on sentencing pregnant women."

I can't believe it. The years charge by and the powers that be are still living in the dark ages responding with reviews, discussions, investigations, taking things further but never any positive action.

Janey Starling, co-director of 'Level Up' which campaigns for gender justice, said: "It's long overdue to end the practice of sentencing pregnant women to custody. When supported in their communities,

they can give their baby the best start in life."

We all know that so --- why don't they? No child should begin his or her life in a prison cell.

******

And then at last I see the figures I have been searching for, in an article in the *Observer* today (October 29th 2023) by Hannah Summers and Nic Murray.

A headline about **pregnant women in jail** is such a rarity that I count these two journalists as my heroes.

Figures published by the Ministry of Justice show that there were 194 pregnant women recorded as being in prison in England and Wales between April 2022 and March 2023.

And 34% of these women were being held on remand awaiting trial. There were 44 births to women in custody and these women are seven times more likely to suffer a stillbirth than those in the general population.

Obviously there are more calls for this practice to end but, take it from me, no-one is listening.

****

YOUNG OFFENDERS

I have written at length about the treatment of young offenders in my previous books but I think we need to see what is happening in 2023. Have conditions improved in Young Offenders Institutes? Well let's find out.

Here is the report from the Chief Inspector of Prisons.

HM Chief Inspector of Prisons for England and Wales Annual Report 2022–23

For the period 1 April 2022 to 31 March 2023

Presented to Parliament pursuant to Section 5A of the Prison Act 1952.

Ordered by the House of Commons to be printed on 5 July 2023

Young offender institutions (YOIs) are juvenile establishments that hold children under the age of 18. Other establishments hold young adults over the age of 18. Juvenile establishments are inspected annually.

"Outcome of previous recommendations in the YOIs reported on in 2022–23:

- *67% of our previous main/key concern recommendations in the area of safety had been achieved and 33% had not been achieved*

- *50% of our previous main/key concern recommendations in the area of care had been achieved and 50% had not been achieved*

- *60% of our previous main/key concern recommendations in the area of purposeful activity had been achieved and 40% had not been achieved*

- *57% of our previous main/key concern recommendations in the area of resettlement had been achieved and 43% had not been achieved."*

The report goes on to paint a picture where there had been a few improvements to life in these institutes but where there are still too many which fail abysmally in their treatment of vulnerable children.

Daily life is generally not child-friendly.

"Accommodation at many YOIs was not designed for children; in particular, the very large living units at Werrington and Wetherby were institutional and did not support effective relationships or behaviour management. The lack of private rooms at Cookham Wood and Feltham also hindered children's access to interventions and activities.

Cleanliness had improved across most sites; most notably at Parc; communal areas had been kept clean, equipment was in good condition and well maintained, and staff encouraged and helped children to keep their cells clean. Parc seems to do quite well in most areas.

But most children continued to eat all their meals alone in their cells. Again the exception was Parc where children enjoyed eating their meals together, and staff sat or ate with them at mealtimes. Feltham had also started doing this on a rota, although most meals continued to be eaten in cell.

The introduction of laptops for every child was a very good initiative. YOIs had moved towards an electronic system for children to make applications for day-to-day services, and the laptops were set up to provide helpful information, make applications or raise complaints, and enable children to check their prison shop spending themselves without relying on staff to do it."

There were reports on health and on diversity in various places but the most worrying area is that of **Purposeful activity.**

Too much time is still spent locked up in their cells. The report says that *"After five Independent Reviews of Progress (IRPs) during the year, we found that reasonable progress had been made against only one of five recommendations about the time children spent out of their cells. No YOI met our expectation that children should be unlocked for 10 hours a day. Parc came the closest with between eight and 11 hours on weekdays. Regimes were more limited at the other four YOIs, offering up to 6.5 hours unlocked on weekdays at Feltham, six hours at Cookham Wood and Wetherby, and 5.5 hours at Werrington. Weekends were worse at all five sites with an average of between three and six hours out of cell on Saturdays and Sundays.*

However, delivery of these regimes was inconsistent and some children experienced very little time out of cell. Staff difficulties at all sites, except Parc, resulted in regime curtailments that restricted children's time unlocked. This often affected the evening and weekend activities that supported relationship-building with staff and peers, and children's well-being. Conflicts between children could further limit time out of cell."

PHYSICAL EDUCATION

Most children had regular access to physical education and time in the fresh air, but opportunities to visit on-site libraries were not as good.

EDUCATION

Parc had maintained the very effective education it had provided during the pandemic and was assessed by Estyn as delivering excellent outcomes for children. In contrast, Ofsted assessed outcomes at Feltham as requiring improvement and at Werrington as inadequate. Children at Werrington could only attend a maximum of 15 hours of education weekly and this was further reduced by late arrival at lessons. So some improvement from a very low bar.

But then we see this.

On 27th April 2023 the Chief Inspector of Prisons issued an **Urgent Notification** to the Secretary of State for Justice demanding immediate action to improve the conditions at the YOI **Cookham Wood** in Kent. This means that he has to reply within 28 days.

Apparently children felt unsafe here and were resorting to carrying weapons. Many had been made by the boys who had scavenged metal from kettles and the like. The prison was dirty and uncared for and the staff were exhausted and felt unsupported by senior managers.

Charlie Taylor, the Chief Inspector of Prisons said: "Many of these children have committed serious crimes and have rightly been detained. Nevertheless, they are still children, many of whom have come from difficult backgrounds. They ought to be receiving education and support to make better choices in the future, supporting their rehabilitation and growth into adulthood so they leave custody in a better position than they entered it. We spoke to boys who'd had almost no human contact at all in days, and who had resorted to trying to stick up photos of home with toothpaste on the walls of the tiny cells that became their whole world. Such treatment of children is appalling. This is a scandal and it cannot be allowed to continue."

Prisons Minister Damian Hinds said: "Cookham Wood is home to some of society's most troubled children, many with violent convictions, but the situation there is completely unacceptable as it is preventing us from helping these young offenders turn their backs on crime.

"That is why we have already appointed a new governor to provide stronger leadership and started a review into how children were being separated to prevent violence but it is clear further action is needed."

Then I see that on the 6th October 2023 Staff working at Cookham Wood, are calling on the government to allow them to use PAVA spray to better protect themselves from these violent children. Apparently in 2018 the government announced that PAVA spray would be rolled out to all male category A to D prisons but a decision on its further use was still being considered. Judith Feline, a former governor at Maidstone prison and ex-prison officer at Cookham Wood, was undecided on whether PAVA spray was the solution to cutting violence.

She told BBC South East: "I don't know whether PAVA is the solution. I have seen it used in the adult estate and it has a pretty nasty effect on you, because your eyes run and it's very sore, but it stops you doing whatever you are doing.

"There are all sorts of issues using that on children. They might be violent young men but they are kids, it's a very difficult decision to make," she added.

A Ministry of Justice spokesperson said: "We continue to provide additional support to HMYOI Cookham Wood and the new governor, appointed earlier this year, is building on progress already made to reduce violence and the number of children being kept apart."

"The safety and welfare of those children in our care and our staff is paramount and we're committed to improving safety across all our sites which is why we are currently considering all the evidence before making a decision on the further roll-out of PAVA."

I really cannot believe they would use this incapacitating spray on young people in prison.

As Wikipedia says it "primarily affects the eyes, causing closure and severe pain. The pain to the eyes is reported to be greater than that caused by CS. The effectiveness rate is very high once PAVA gets into the eyes."

The treatment of our young people in prison is, in many cases, inhumane.

****

Then on the 17th November 2023 I receive the most recent Ofsted report on **Oakhill Secure Training Centre.** It was published today on the GOV. UK website. I have signed up to receive these reports of inspections and this one took place from the 2nd to the 6th October 2023. The lead Inspector was Lisa Summers, Ofsted, His Majesty's Inspector.

Oakhill provides accommodation for up to 80 children, male and female, aged 12 to 19 years, who are serving a custodial sentence or who are remanded to custody by the courts. There were 59 children resident at the time of the inspection, 57 boys and two girls.

Why were they there? What had they done to warrant being locked up? What was their background? What sort of support were they receiving before being sent here? And two girls? How do they get on in a place such as this?

Well I don't know the answers to any of these questions but I do know that at the inspection in 2021 the centre was deemed to be inadequate in all aspects but one which was the children's health. So let's see what has improved since then.

Well the general summary was that overall experiences and progress of children and young people requires improvement to be good but the education and learning is now good and the health has continued to be good. .

But children's resettlement, how children are helped and protected and also the effectiveness of leaders and managers all require improvements to be good.

But this is good to hear.

"Across the centre, there is a tangible change in culture, with children being recognised and treated as children first and foremost."

Yes well that seems sensible.

But then we are on to the most common problem everywhere.

"Despite significant efforts made by staff and managers to ensure that children receive good-quality care and have positive experiences, staff shortages and changes have compromised the quality of care that children receive."

This is a long and detailed report and it is obvious that there is improvement in certain areas but children are still being locked in their rooms for too long, some children do not get the same rewards for good behaviour as others due to lack of facilities which results in apathy and the dining room is not used enough which, as we have heard before, would encourage more socialised behaviour.

The children still need better support in order to improve their reading skills and the report states that they can *"Improve children's quality of care by providing timely conflict resolution to increase opportunities for more children to mix with their peers when it is safe for them to do so; – helping staff to feel confident and to intervene in disputes between children at an early stage to prevent escalation to violence and the need for physical restraint."*

They can also *"Improve children's resettlement by helping to prepare them to return to the community through the delivery of high-quality interventions, key working, high quality release on temporary license (ROTL) and regular family days."*

And then when they are released back into their previous lives how much support is there waiting for them I wonder?

Well if you have read this far you will know the answer to that question. Every single chapter describes the lack of concern for our young people by this government.

Young people in prison are no exception.

****

Then today (21st November 2023) Charlie Taylor, comments in *The Guardian* on two reports from his inspectorate which paint a "bleak picture" of youth custody in England and Wales. His main concern is that prisons holding children are "significantly more violent" than jails holding adult men and most fail to deliver "one meaningful conversation with a child each week."

Well I have already seen and commented on Cookham Wood and Oakhill but he also mentions Werrington YOI. The inspection of Werrington, also just published, found that serious disorder had increased by 76% over the past year, with multiple incidents requiring the deployment of national resources. This included groups of boys trying to smash through doors to get to other children.

He said that despite the government spending £300,000 a year for every child in custody, levels of violence and self-harm are rising across the youth prison estate in England and Wales.

But he urged the government not to allow the use of pepper spray on incarcerated children saying it "risks increasing rather than reducing hostility."

And again this is important to note. The average population of children and young people held in STCs and YOIs was 434 in 2022–23, compared with 939 in 2015–16 so numbers have gone down.

But the crumbling prison estate, the lack of experienced staff, and the lack of educational resources still means that many young offenders can go without any face to face contact for days on end.

****

How do the police treat our children? We are all very aware of the misogyny they show to women and the racism that exists especially in the Met, as was found in the report by Louise Casey in March this year when she found the Met to be "institutionally racist, misogynistic and homophobic."

There is an article in the *Times* today (23rd November 2023) by Ali Mitib about the practice of strip- searching children without "appropriate consent".

You might have read about the 15 year old black girl who was wrongly accused of carrying cannabis at school and had been strip-searched by police during her period. This was three years ago. A report this year by Dame Rachel de Souza, the Children's Commissioner, found that **children as young as eight were being stopped and strip-searched**

by police. More than half of these took place without an appropriate adult present.

A senior paediatrician has called for these kind of searches, those without an appropriate adult present, to be banned. Professor Andrew Bush writing in the 'Archives of Diseases in Childhood', which is the official journal of the Royal College of Paediatrics and Child Health, states that police should be subject to the same protocols as doctors. Unless they can justify their actions to an independent panel **"they should be dismissed and have to sign the sex-offender's register."**

Yes, he says that, "As with an adult, removing someone's clothing without consent is sexual abuse".

So once again we hear of people in authority treating children as though they are of no consequence. This leaves me with a continuation of the sense of burning anger which causes me to write this book.

****

*"He who opens a school door,
closes a prison."*

Victor Hugo

****

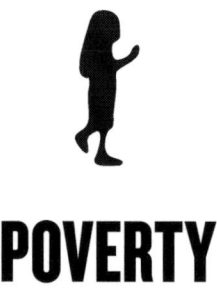

POVERTY

So what do we mean by the word poverty?

According to the House of Commons Library, poverty in the UK is defined in terms of disposable household income (income after adding on benefits and deducting direct taxes). However, poverty may be defined in different ways and there is no single, universally accepted definition. Two commonly used measures of poverty based on disposable income are:

- Relative low income: This refers to people living in households with income below 60% of the median in that year.

- Absolute low income: This refers to people living in households with income below 60% of median income **in a base year**, usually 2010/11. This measurement is adjusted for inflation. Median income is the point at which half of households have lower income and half have higher income. Income can be measured before or after housing costs are deducted. The 'Joseph Rowntree Foundation' (JRF) reported that in 2021, about 1 in 5 (20%) of people in the UK lived in poverty.

- Poverty means not being able to heat your home, pay your rent, or buy the essentials for your children.

Then I see a charity focused on children in London called 'The Childhood Trust'. This is a charity which funds the delivery of youth projects and services that support thousands of disadvantaged children and young people in London every year.

On their website they state that:

"We fund the delivery of grassroots projects, run volunteer community support programmes, and produce original research and advocacy to improve the life chances of disadvantaged children in the capital and build capacity in London's child support sector. Our growing community of corporate supporters, philanthropists, and donors combined with our strong relationships with established children's charities make us well-equipped to direct resources to London's most economically disadvantaged and isolated communities."

Their London Child Poverty Report written in 2021 by this Trust makes upsetting reading. This is a long report detailing the problems and also making some firm recommendations. I will just highlight a few points made in the Executive Summary.

"London has the highest child poverty rate in England. While other cities in Europe have seen their rates of childhood poverty decline, London's has been increasing for the past five years. As one of the most expensive cities in the world, low levels of household income are compounded by extremely high housing, transportation and childcare costs.

Additionally, cuts to benefits and tax credits as part of a larger restructuring of the British welfare state have contributed to higher levels of poverty.

"The "decade of austerity" ushered in by the coalition government beginning in 2010 has been one of the greatest factors in terms of increasing child poverty. Cuts have been made to benefits, local authorities, family support services and countless other social programmes; nearly half of London councils' youth services have been slashed. Despite this, demand for such services is ever present and food bank usage in London has increased over 17-fold between 2011/2012 and 2019/2020. The policy has suppressed household incomes and hit the poor the hardest. In the capital, one in six parents have children in food insecurity. Food insecurity is when one is unable to access reliable, sufficient, affordable, nutritious food."

This a dreadful indictment on government policies.

The 'Child Poverty Action Group' reports that the most recently-published 'Household Below Average Income' figures say that there were **4.2 million children** living in poverty in the UK in 2021-22. That's 29 % of children, or **nine in a classroom of 30**.

They go on to say that work does not provide a guaranteed route out of poverty in the UK. 71% of children growing up in poverty live in a **household where at least one person works**.

And note this: Between 1998 and 2003 reducing child poverty was made a priority under a Labour government - with a comprehensive strategy and investment in children - and the number of children in poverty fell by 600,000.

This just proves that **Nelson Mandela** is absolutely correct when he says that **"Overcoming poverty is not a task of charity, it is an act of justice. Like Slavery and Apartheid, poverty is not natural. It is man-made and it can be overcome and eradicated by the actions of human beings. Sometimes it falls on a generation to be great. YOU can be that great generation. Let your greatness blossom."**

But everything falls on deaf ears for it also reveals the inadequacies of this government as they have allowed so many people to suffer for so long. I am horrified by the response of the government to the hardship of so many people.

When so many charities are calling for sweeping reforms of the welfare system, the uplifting of Universal Credit, further food security and access to healthier foods, more subsidised transport and more social housing, plus a change in employment practices such as zero-hour contracts and part-time jobs laws what does this government do?

They decide to end free Transport for London travel for under 18s which will mean that many disadvantaged students will be unable to travel to school this autumn. Then they respond to the inevitable increase in the crime of shoplifting in a draconian and heartless way.

Akiko Hart is the interim director of 'Liberty' and he writes in the *Guardian* on the 12th October 2023 that one in ten young people have shoplifted to cope with the rise in the cost of living. And what are the most shoplifted items? Calpol and formula milk.

So the government is utterly appalled by this and is going to increase the use of facial recognition technology to track shoplifters and stop them once and for all. As Mr. Hart says **"this feels like an attempt to criminalise poverty."**

Chris Philp the policing minister is setting this up and it will be a national shoplifting data which can be used by police and retailers nationwide. Such a database could include the passport photos of 45 million adults in the country.

But actually this kind of facial recognition technology, which allows police forces to identify and track anyone they choose, regardless of suspicion, is already happening. Philp acknowledged a few weeks ago that all 45 police forces are currently using it.

Did you know that? Well I certainly didn't and many people are calling for a ban on this already. John Lewis has decided not to continue using facial recognition in their stores and last week, dozens of cross-party MPs and peers joined calls for an immediate stop to the use of live facial recognition surveillance by police and private companies.

Then we hear from Matt Dathan who is the Home Affairs Editor of the *Sunday Times*. He writes on the 22nd October that there is to be a summit meeting in Downing Street where more plans to stop shoplifting will be unveiled by police chiefs.

These plans will include a dedicated national unit – Operational Opal – that will investigate shoplifting cases from an organised crime perspective.

The "zero-tolerance" plan will also see police forces sign up to a new commitment to attend the scene of every shoplifting incident reported to them that involves a threat of violence to store and security employees.

Wow. Where are those police going to come from?

But if all else fails you are allowed to make a citizen's arrest. OK? If you see someone stealing something from a store Chris Philp says:

"Where it's safe to do so I would encourage that to be used, because if you do just let people walk in and take stuff and walk out without proper challenge, including potentially a physical challenge, then it will just escalate."

Then he does acknowledge that there are not enough police because he goes on to say that "While I want the faster and better police response, they can't be everywhere so I would still think about stores setting that up in some cases."

That actually sounds extremely dangerous to me and if this is all they can come up with then I despair.

As Mr. Hart goes on to say "The challenges that shoplifting creates are best addressed by understanding the impact rising costs and poverty are having on people across the country who are struggling to pay their bills and feed their children. Basic foods like bread, butter and cheese have risen in price by more than a third in the past year, alongside skyrocketing energy, housing and fuel costs.

"Far from keeping us safe, spy tech used on the general public undermines the rights and freedoms that protect us from state control and discrimination. The safest thing for everyone is to ban facial recognition technology."

And Alex Norris, the shadow policing minister, said government officials have gutted neighbourhood police forces, leaving shops more vulnerable to crime.

"Rather than offering serious suggestions to get police back on the beat, the minister is inviting even more violence against shop workers by calling for citizen's arrests, while making pie-in-the-sky promises about databases when the Tories have still failed to upgrade the police national computer" he said.

"The Tories are just making it up as they go along but communities are paying the price."

Well yes, all policies seem to be being made on the hoof at the moment. It would appear that due to the significant lack of police due to the vast cuts in public spending we, the general public, are required to step in and do their work for them.

I say, how about following the advice of excellent charities, some of whom I explore below?

****

The 'Child Poverty Action Group'

This is what they say on their website.

"Child Poverty Action Group' works on behalf of the more than one in four children in the UK growing up in poverty. It doesn't have to be like this. We work to understand what causes poverty, the impact it has on children's lives, and how it can be prevented and solved – for good.

"Poverty is not inevitable. It is caused by low wages, inadequate benefits, expensive housing and childcare, and a lack of decently-paid jobs. Drawing on our 50 years of experience and expertise, we devise and promote solutions we know will lift children and families out of poverty. Our vision is of a society free of child poverty, where all children can enjoy a childhood free of financial hardship and have an equal chance in life to reach their full potential."

This is what they say is needed to be done.

Scrap the two-child limit. The two-child limit restricts support in universal credit and tax credits to two children in a family, affecting third or subsequent children born after 6 April 2017. Scrapping the two-child limit would be the most cost-effective way to reduce child poverty. It would lift 250,000 children out of poverty and mean 850,000 children are in less deep poverty.

Abolish the benefit cap. The benefit cap restricts the total amount of support a working-age household can receive from the social security system if they are earning less than the equivalent of 16 hours a week at the minimum wage or not in paid work. 250,000 children live in households affected by the cap. A lone parent with three children is now likely to be capped across most areas of the country, and can be left with as little as £44 a week to live on after paying housing costs.

Raise child benefit by £20 a week per child. Child benefit is a payment made to the main carer of a child, with an amount for each child they care for. It is not means-tested, but if someone in the household earns over £50,000 there is a charge to pay – the high-income child benefit charge (HICBC). Increasing child benefit by £20 a week would see 500,000 children pulled out of poverty.

Roll out universal free school meals across England. (Oh how often do we hear this?) Free school meals refer to the midday meal provided to children across the UK. At the moment, a lot of this provision is means-tested, but in some areas, for some ages of children, there is universal provision. CPAG's analysis shows that 900,000 children in poverty in England do not currently qualify for free school meals."

They also say that a new national childcare strategy should include:

- a high-quality, fully-funded model of the 30-hour free entitlement to childcare available to all families, *regardless of employment status;*

- increased support for children's centres; and

- comprehensive, 8am to 6pm out-of-school and holiday wraparound childcare through extended school days.

- The waiting period for a first payment of universal credit should be reduced to two weeks.

- Attention needs to be paid to second earners. Extending universal credit work allowances to second earners would allow families to keep more of their earnings and escape poverty sooner through work.

They urge the UK government to recommit to ending poverty as a national priority, with a comprehensive strategy and targets.

Well I think all this sounds practical, possible and humane. But I don't think the government has read these recommendations.

****

Because then I read this.

The 'Joseph Rowntree Foundation' has today (October 24th) published a new report entitled '**Destitution in the UK 2023.**'

This is not poverty they are talking about. According to the Cambridge dictionary the word destitute means someone without money, food, a home, or possessions. And a destitute child means a child under the age of eighteen who is in a state of want or suffering due to lack of sufficient food, clothing, shelter, or medical or surgical care.

The research lays out starkly not simply the scale of destitution in this country, but how potently it has spread.

The number of people experiencing destitution in the UK has more than doubled in the last five years.

One million children are now living in destitute homes- a staggering increase of 186% in half a decade.

But the following has an impact on children too of course. This research, which is part of a project that has been monitoring the scale of destitution since 2015, found that almost two-thirds of adults who are in severe poverty have a disabling or long-term health condition and cancer patients going to chemotherapy come home to wear a coat in their freezing homes.

Frances Ryan of the *Guardian* on the 24th October writes .that " 'Destitute' is a term that conjures up the Victorian era – a living standard so sparse, so removed from modern civilisation, that by all rights it should be consigned to the history books. You only have to read through the aching interviews in the JRF study to see what destitution in modern Britain looks like: children wearing their parents' clothes because that's all there is in the wardrobe; eating a banana as a single daytime meal; taking the one permitted toilet roll a week from the local church donation. Gone are the workhouses. Nowadays, we send the poor to sift through charity bins."

Nearly three-quarters of people experiencing destitution are in receipt of social security payments, which the 'Joseph Rowntree Foundation' cites as further evidence of benefit inadequacy. They find that a cash freeze on 'non-protected' benefits such as Universal Credit would save roughly £4.1bn a year. However it warns that this would result in nine million families facing a permanent hit of £460 a year.

As I keep writing I keep thinking it can't get any worse.

But it does. Andrew Cooper, who was the Tory candidate in last week's Tamworth by-election said that jobless parents who are struggling to feed their children while paying for a phone should "fuck off."

Hmmm. Labour won a historic victory in Tamworth with the second highest **ever** Tory-to-**Labour** swing of 23.9% so I don't think that that was an election winning phrase.

Just who on earth are these people and how on earth do they justify using this sort of language?

And also today, 24ᵗʰ October, as we read the report on destitution, we hear that the government is to scrap the ban on banker's bonuses with effect from next week. So instead of only being able to have twice their annual salary as a bonus they will now have as much as anyone wants to give them.

The move has been called 'an insult to working people.'

You won't be surprised to hear that I call it ignorant and callous.

****

And now I write about another charity which is concerned with the poverty of the UK.

This is the 'Trussell Trust'.

The 'Trussell Trust' charity has just conducted their most in-depth study to date on hunger which reveals its causes, impacts and who is affected. It was published in June 2023 and is entitled 'Hunger in the UK'.

This research was produced in partnership with Ipsos and drew on the time and expertise of very many people and other charities and companies. The report is 100 pages long so I can only pick out the more salient facts but it is extremely important.

I begin with this appalling statistic.

Today there are nearly 1,400 Trussell Trust food banks plus an additional 1,172 independent food banks in the UK. **In 2010 there were around 35**.

And food banks in the Trussell Trust network distributed almost three million parcels in the year to April 2023, the most parcels ever distributed in a single year, and a 37% increase on 2021/22

We really need to understand exactly why this should be so.

The forward by Emma Revie states that:-

"More and more people in our society are being left with no option but to turn to a food bank to feed themselves or their family. But as our most in-depth study on hunger to date shows, this is just the tip of the iceberg."

Of course we hear the government say over and over again that if only more and more people could get into work all would be well. They also say that the welfare system and universal benefits are increasing all the time in order to help those on low incomes.

So let us see what the 'Trussell Trust' found out and how it impacts on children first and foremost.

Profiling those who most need foodbanks they found that households with children make up a much larger proportion of those who are food insecure and who turn to food banks than in the general population.

The government again always sites the pandemic and the rise in the cost of living for any increase in the dependency of food banks but the report says:

"The significant impact of the pandemic and the rise in the cost of living must not distract from a longer-term and more pervasive rise in food insecurity and food bank need; **this increase long pre-dates the start of the pandemic.**

" In the five years between 2017/18 and 2022/23, the number of emergency food parcels which the 'Trussell Trust' network of food banks had to provide more than doubled, with a similar trend of rising need seen by other providers of food aid in the UK."

And to emphasise the tip of the iceberg comment they say:-

"More than two thirds of those experiencing food insecurity have not received food aid. Food bank use therefore does not represent the entirety of need across the country, but rather those who have accessed this form of support – many more people appear to be facing serious hardship without such help."

And then of course all families using food banks affect children.

"Families with children are at a high risk of food insecurity. Nearly half (47%) of all households experiencing food insecurity include children under the age of 16."

And then we see how the whole set-up of the welfare state is failing people and also how being employed, as others have already said, does not necessarily mean you have enough money to live on. They say:-

"Three main factors combine to prevent people from having sufficient income to avoid food insecurity, and leave them having to turn to food banks:-

• The design and delivery of the social security system.

• Work which does not provide sufficient protection from financial hardship.

- Difficulty accessing suitable jobs, especially for disabled people, people with caring responsibilities and parents (especially mothers)."

The report goes on:-

"The number of people supported through Universal Credit doubled from three million in March 2020 to more than six million in March 2021. (This was due to the pandemic). In many ways, the system met the huge increase in need very successfully, processing claims and ensuring support reached most people faster than many had feared. However, the inadequacy of the level of support provided, the design issues within the social security system including the five-week wait for the first payment, and the hardship these insufficiencies created, were also exposed.

"Analysis in 2021 showed that increases in claims for Universal Credit are associated with rises in the numbers of people who also need to turn to a food bank. **At the point that the Covid-19 pandemic took hold in the UK in March 2020, the level of support provided by the UK social security system had been eroded by a series of cuts and freezes over the previous decade."**

Then we hear about pay.

"The fundamental reason most people are referred to food banks is that their income is too low for them to be able to afford the essentials we all need in life. The most significant driver of this is design and delivery of the social security system.

"Paid work is not always a solution with one in five (20%) people referred to food banks in the 'Trussell Trust' network being from a working household, as low pay and insecure jobs still leave them with insufficient income to afford the essentials. Others would like to work but find that jobs are inaccessible, especially for disabled people, people with caring responsibilities and people – especially women – with children."

And how many people realise or even think about the problems that can be had trying to access the internet and the importance of that? They say:-

"Not being able to access the internet can also exacerbate poverty, as often the best financial offers and access for goods and services are found online, as are various application routes for additional support and grants. We found that people referred to food banks who do not have access to the internet are less likely to have applied for, or received, any of the local crisis support (23%) than people with access to the internet (28%) Children's education also tends to assume families have internet access, with children needing to go online to complete homework or other educational activities."

Then there is the complete lack of understanding about the cost of living essentials.

"Research by the 'Trussell Trust' and the 'Joseph Rowntree Foundation' has calculated that the cost of essentials (food, utilities, and vital household goods), is currently at least £120 a week for a single adult and £200 for a couple. However, the basic rate of benefits is far lower than this, as are the incomes of people referred to food banks in the 'Trussell Trust' network. The average income after housing costs for those referred to a food bank is just £87 amongst single adults living on their own or with children, and £145 amongst couples with or without children"

But "for most people referred to food banks in the 'Trussell Trust' network, the design and delivery of the social security system are major contributors to their inability to afford the essentials."

The whole welfare system would appear to be completely inadequate and non-user-friendly.

a) First, the process for applying can be confusing and there is a lack of accessible information about what people are entitled to.

b) Secondly, when people do apply there are difficulties claiming benefits quickly and consistently, this is particularly the case for Personal Independence Payments (PIP) for people affected by disability, or a long-term mental or physical health condition.

c) Thirdly, even when secured, the level of payments provides insufficient income to meet essential needs.

d) Finally, in many cases, unaffordable reductions may be taken off each month, further reducing people's income.

"Cuts and freezes to benefit payments over the last decade have led to a large reduction in the purchasing power of benefits relative to the rising cost of living. In 2022, there was the greatest fall in the value of the basic rate of unemployment benefits since the start of annual uprating fifty years ago.

The low level of benefit payments is a key contributor to people needing to access food banks as they are left without enough money to afford the essentials

A variety of research and evidence demonstrates that providing more income via the social security system can reduce destitution. The positive effect of the £20 uplift to Universal Credit between April 2020 and October 2021 has been well-documented and led to reductions in both food insecurity and child poverty."

Indeed we were all aware of that and we were horrified when it was stopped.

Then the government will say, and does indeed say very often when faced with any criticism, that they have handed out cost of living payments for those who need it so they should all be OK.

But the report states that:-

"After each Cost of Living Payment was distributed in July and November, there was a short-term reduction in need at food banks in the 'Trussell Trust' network.

Both of these impacts were significant but short-lived, demonstrating that increasing incomes does reduce the need for food banks, but one-off payments cannot make a lasting difference when people's regular income (from social security and from work) is just too low cover the essentials."

I would have thought that this was obvious.

"Work should provide reliable protection from destitution, but it is clear that for a significant number of people this is not the case."

"30% of people in paid work referred to food banks in the 'Trussell Trust' network are in insecure work."

"Childcare presents a significant barrier to work, as has also been found in a wide range of previous research. Excluding people who are not working due to a health condition, one in seven (14%) people in non-working households with children cited a lack of affordable childcare as the reason they were out of work.

"Almost all (91%) were women. One in three working mothers have lost work or hours due to childcare.

"Parents – particularly women – discussed the challenges in finding flexible and secure work which they could fit around childcare commitments."

And then there are health issues.

"One participant described how their son had been diagnosed with a rare health condition meaning that they needed to stop work temporarily while they cared for their child. This had significantly impacted their financial situation."

Well, the above is just a small flavour of this detailed and well-researched report.

They conclude by saying:-

"In one of the richest economies in the world, one in seven people are experiencing food insecurity, many of them going hungry due to lack of money.

"The drivers of hunger are complex and multi-faceted, with debt, insecure work, social isolation and adverse life events exacerbating financial hardship, but **it is clear that an inadequate social security system is the most significant driver of food bank need**.

"That is why introducing an 'Essentials Guarantee' into our social security system – a change to legislation which would ensure that the basic rate of Universal Credit is always enough for people to afford the essentials – would take us a significant distance down the road towards a UK without the need for the food banks. This report demonstrates the urgent need for this policy change and the importance of it being supported by all who are committed to making the UK a country without the need for food banks."

Meanwhile our children go hungry to school.

****

This does not help either.

NO FAULT EVICTION

The ban on "no-fault" evictions in England will be indefinitely delayed until after the court system is reformed, the government has just announced. (24th October 2023)

After the court system is reformed? How many decades do we have to wait for that?

The Renters Reform Bill, promised in the Tories' 2019 election manifesto, was debated in the Commons for the first time on Monday 23rd. October. 2023.

The proposed law, which will ban no-fault "Section 21" evictions, was first published in May.

But Housing Secretary Michael Gove said yesterday that it was "vital" to update the courts first. Mr. Gove has told Conservative MPs that the ban cannot be enacted before a series of improvements are made in the court system, which is used by some landlords to reclaim possession of their homes.

So what is this all about?

Landlords can currently evict tenants who are not on fixed-term contracts without giving a reason, under housing legislation known as Section 21.

After receiving a Section 21 notice, tenants have two months before their landlord can apply for a court order to evict them.

Under the government's new bill however, all tenancies would become "rolling" contracts with no fixed end date.

Labour accused the government of kicking the much-delayed proposals into the "long grass", arguing legal reforms would "take years" to complete and put thousands of renters at risk of eviction.

We really need to go searching in that long grass.

Indeed this is going to continue to cause much hardship as so many people have said that it took them longer than two months to find somewhere else to live.

Indeed according to annual government figures released last week the number of households in England who became homeless or were at risk of homelessness increased by nearly 7% in the year to March. There was a 23% increase in people at risk of homelessness because of a section 21 "no fault eviction".

'Shelter', the housing charity which has co-ordinated a letter from 30 organisations to Rishi Sunak, wrote that its research suggested a renter is evicted every three minutes in England under the no-fault rule.

"This dire lack of security disproportionately impacts the people we represent," 'Shelter' said.

Its letter pointed out that "poor and insecure housing makes people physically sick, and has a well-documented, negative impact on their mental health".

It added: "It causes social isolation and financial hardship, and traps people in cycles of poverty, struggle and uncertainty that are difficult, sometimes impossible, to break."

The letter said scrapping no-fault evictions should be "at the heart" of the government's plans, warning that renters "cannot wait any longer".

"Together we are calling on the government to commit to progressing the Renters Reform Bill this parliament, and to pass it into law as promised in the party's manifesto."

Signatories include 'Child Poverty Action Group', 'Citizens Advice',' Liberty', the' Centre for Mental Health and Disability Rights UK.'

Well the progress of this bill continues at a snail's pace. The '**Property Rescue'** website states this:-

"You probably already know that the Queen's Speech in 2022 committed to a Renters' Reform Bill being passed in 2022-23. The bill was delayed due to disruptions caused by changes of government. The Renters' Reform Bill finally arrived in the House of Commons in May 2023 after the King's Coronation. Currently, the Renters' Reform Bill is at 'Second Reading' stage. When will the Renters Reform Bill become law?

"While no official date has been confirmed by the government, we estimate that the Renters Reform Bill will come into law on 1st October 2024. Once it becomes law, it will initially only affect new tenancies. Pre-existing tenancies will be included 12 months later."

So October 2025 then. Possibly. The word 'urgent' is simply not in the vocabulary of this government.

And of course the impact on children is horrendous.

In 2020 'Shelter' said that 183 children lost their homes every single day - that›s enough children to fill two double-decker buses. **A child becomes homeless in Britain every eight minutes according to their findings.**

Today 2023 new research from 'Shelter' shows at least 271,000 people are recorded as homeless in England, including **123,000 children.**

Then I read another shocking statistic which is that **at a school in the borough of Southwark, 81% of their children are homeless.** Mothers of children at the school in Peckham gathered together one morning in December to talk to Megan Agnew, a feature writer for *the Sunday Times*. It is heart-breaking. So many children are in temporary accommodation and some do not know where they will return to at the end of the school day. Often they are moved around with little notice and so end up travelling miles to school which is their one constant, safe place. Many are sleeping in one room with their family and one eight year old girl describes how she puts up posters and maps on the walls to hide the mould and damp in her room, but that she gets so cold that she becomes ill and unable to go to school. Obviously this sort of situation has an enormous negative effect on the mental wellbeing of children. As Ms. Agnew reports, "some withdraw, others become nervous and others become enraged, angry all the time." Some of the mothers were weeping as they told their stories.

In 2011 there were 48,000 households in England in temporary accommodation. By this year, 2023, that number had risen to over 104,000, the highest since records began in 1998. (Ministry of Housing, Communities & Local Government.)

And then we read this and so we now understand. A report in the *Telegraph* suggested Tory MPs who owned rental properties were considering rebelling against the government over the bill. Because surprise, surprise research by campaign group "38 Degrees' found 87 MPs earned an income from letting out residential property, of which 68 were Conservatives - about one fifth of Tory MPs. The passing of this bill would make life much more difficult for them and that cannot be allowed to happen.

The Liberal Democrats have called on all 68 Tory MPs who are landlords to reveal if they have ever used a Section 21 notice against their tenants "in order to have greater transparency over why they may oppose the ban on them."

And just today (1st December) LBC declares that they have seen figures which suggest that 12,500 families will be issued with no-fault eviction notices between now and Christmas Day.

A 'Shelter' solicitor, Kirsty Almond says the rate of evictions and the suffering is the worst she's ever seen in her 15 years in this 'Shelter' job, with incomes no longer covering rent and mortgage rises. The last year has seen nearly 40% more section 21 no-fault evictions in England.

The 'Renters' Reform Coalition' a campaign group that has been pushing for a ban, called the announcement a "last-minute concession to keep the Conservative Party together".

Campaign manager Tom Darling said: "The idea that some ill-defined 'court reform' must happen before section 21 no-fault evictions can end is absurd."

Absurd? Everything about this government is increasingly absurd and it is young children who are bearing the brunt. Child poverty alone is estimated to be costing the economy £39 billion a year due to the extra strain on public services and future unemployment.

****

And today (6th November) the UK is told off by the United Nations special rapporteur on extreme poverty and human rights. I can't believe it. It is humiliating and appalling that we should hear these words from such a respected organisation.

Olivier De Schutter, the UN's poverty envoy has said that the UK Government is violating international law. Credit payments of £85 a week for single adults over 25 were "grossly insufficient" and described the UK's main welfare system as a "leaking bucket".

Five years ago, his predecessor, Philip Alston, accused the Conservative government of the "systematic immiseration of a significant part of the British population". Well the Conservatives didn't like that at all.

And they will like this even less as today Olivier De Schutter says, "Things have got a lot worse."

Speaking to *The Guardian*, De Schutter said: **"It's simply not acceptable that we have more than a fifth of the population in a rich country such as the UK at risk of poverty today,"** as he referred to data showing 14.4 million people lived in relative poverty in 2021-22.

"The policies in place are not working or not protecting people in poverty, and much more needs to be done for these people to be protected."

Absolutely we all say Amen to that and we have been saying this for years.

He added that the UK had signed an international covenant that created a duty to provide a level of social protection which ensured an adequate standard of living but that this was being broken.

Well I never knew about this covenant. But here it is.

The International Covenant on Economic, Social and Cultural Rights is a multilateral treaty adopted by the United Nations General Assembly on 16th December 1966 through General Assembly Resolution 2200A, and came into force on 3rd January 1976. It is part of the International Bill of Human Rights, along with the Universal Declaration of Human Rights and the International Covenant on Civil and Political Rights.

The rights include labour rights, the right to health, the right to education, and the right to an adequate standard of living.

So there we go. Has this present government read all of this?

De Schutter explained that: "If you look at the price of housing, electricity, the very high levels of inflation for food items over the past couple of years, I believe that the £85 a week for adults is too low to protect people from poverty, and that is in violation of article nine of the international covenant on economic, social (and cultural) rights. That is what human rights law says."

So we are breaking this covenant. He is due to visit the UK this week. Well it was fireworks night last weekend but look out for a few more fireworks during his visit.

And I receive an email from the 'Childhood Trust' today (5th December) highlighting the increase of child poverty in working households in London and displaying a film in which Dr.Olivier De Schutter re-iterates his concern about higher inflation rates causing so much poverty.

****

Then there is a report just out by the charity 'Pregnant then Screwed' which says that the majority of mothers who reduce their maternity leave do so because they are struggling with money.

One in 10 mothers are forced to go back to work within four months of having a child due to being unable to afford to stop working for longer, the report found.

Joeli Brearley, 'Pregnant Then Screwed's founder and chief executive, said: "We have some of the lowest rates of parental leave pay in the world. National minimum wage is the legal minimum a person should be paid, yet new mothers are meant to survive on less than half of this amount for 33 weeks, whilst their outgoings remain the same. And, of course, the cost of living crisis is exacerbating this issue."

Ms. Brearley explained the "perinatal period is critically important" to both the mother and the child's health and welfare as she warned everyone should be "deeply concerned" about the "degeneration and a degradation" of this important time.

"Simultaneously, and I would argue not unrelated, NHS data from August 2022-March 2023 showed an 8 per cent increase in new mothers accessing support for mental health services on the NHS," she added.

"We have also seen an increase in infant mortality in the UK. Poverty has a significant impact on the risk of stillbirth and death during infancy. Ultimately, it is a false economy to not pay parental leave at a rate at which families can survive and thrive."

And so we see further neglect and ignorance from an uncaring government and it is once again up to a charity to bring this to light.

****

Then I see ex-prime minister Gordon Brown has linked up with Amazon to set up a new charity called Multibank. First established 14 months ago in Scotland and then in Manchester, four new multibanks are set to launch in 2024 including in London, the Midlands and Wales, with the idea that there will be multibanks in different parts of the country by the end of next year.

Speaking to the *Evening Standard,* Mr Brown spoke passionately about the extreme levels of poverty he sees. He said: "The level of poverty is something I never expected to see again in my lifetime. The last time I saw this sort of poverty was growing up in a mining, industrial town where there was a great deal of social housing and a great deal of distress. I thought we would never go back to those days again."

A multibank is not just a food bank, but a baby bank, a bedding bank, a clothing bank, a toiletries bank and a furnishings bank. They secure products from about 30 companies, with about half supplied by Amazon out of defunct items and product returns and then work through hundreds of partner charities to supply these essential goods to families in need — who in turn have been referred by social workers, health visitors, schools and food banks.

As we have seen this is absolutely vital to all those families affected so badly by the cost of living crises.

There are so many people working so hard to help those who are living in circumstances not dreamt of just a few years ago.

Zarach is a charity which concentrates on supplying beds and mattresses to those in need.

It was founded in 2017. Zarach has witnessed an enormous increase in the demand for beds over the last 12 months, with 31% of families giving the reason as mental health issues while 23% are victims of domestic abuse.

In a recent report published by Barnardo's, researchers found that 894,000 children in the UK were without a proper bed, and were having to share with family members or sleep on the floor.

In polling collected by YouGov, 20% of children surveyed felt tired at school and 13% struggled during physical activities, while one in 12 parents said their children were "tired all the time" due to not having their own bed to sleep in.

In order to identify families struggling with a lack of available bedding, Zarach has formed close relationships with over 500 schools that provide them with a referral. After conducting a home visit, volunteers deliver a bed frame, duvet, mattress, pillows, pyjamas and a hygiene kit to their property within eight days.

I have mentioned this charity in my previous books '**Beneath the Bluster'** and again in '**Behind the Headlines'**.

****

And as we enter the New Year an article by James Tapper of the *Guardian* states that charities have warned that there has been a dramatic rise in the number of homeless young people in the UK since Christmas.

The New Horizon Youth Centre in London said a record number of young people had asked it for help in the first week of January. 2024. 'Roundabout' in Sheffield and YMCA Trinity, which operates in Cambridgeshire and Suffolk, also reported increases.

A coalition of 120 charities has come together under the banner #PlanForThe136k – which refers to an estimate that there were 136,000 homeless young people in 2023 – to call on the government to create a national strategy to end youth homelessness."

But Rishi Sunak, when asked in an interview whether he lay awake at night worrying about the inequality of the economy and the plight of those living in poverty, replied "No".

****

"Poverty is the worst form of violence."

Mahatma Gandhi,

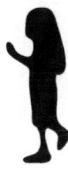

REFUGEE CHILDREN

The treatment of asylum seekers by this government continues to be inhumane, cruel and in many instances, against international law. Suella Braverman, the Home Secretary, (October 2023) uses language which promotes division and hate and she, plus other Ministers including the PM, continue to label all asylum seekers as illegal migrants. Those who understand the situation keep saying that there is no such thing as an illegal asylum seeker but to no avail. The small boats dangerous fiasco could be stopped tomorrow by building an assessment centre in France, training asylum assessors at top speed and then allowing those whose applications are successful (which will be about 80% in total) to travel here on safe and legal routes as is the case with Ukranian refugees. We would then benefit from their skills base and taxes rather than have the burden of out-of-control ever-rising costs.

At the moment all refugees are being treated like criminals, they are being locked up in disgusting conditions and are being denied full and proper access to lawyers. And one refugee on the barge Bibby Stockholm in Dorset has just committed suicide.

But it is the treatment of child refugees which concerns me here and, as in other sectors and as noted in previous chapters, the cruelty, neglect and ignorance is paramount.

First of all we need to deal with a few facts. The Refugee Council states it loudly and clearly! They state that:-

"There is no such thing as an 'illegal' or 'bogus' asylum seeker. Under international law, anyone has the right to apply for asylum in any country that has signed the 1951 Convention and to remain there until the authorities have assessed their claim."

They talk about safe and legal routes:-

"It is recognised in the 1951 Convention that people fleeing persecution may have to use irregular means in order to escape and claim asylum in another country – there is no legal way to travel to the UK for the specific purpose of seeking asylum."

And they state that:-

"The 1951 Refugee Convention guarantees everybody the right to apply for asylum. It has saved millions of lives. No country has ever withdrawn from it."

They also state that there is no international law which says that refugees must claim asylum in the first country they reach.

They are working tirelessly to support these children in any way they can and they say that: "Many of the children we support have endured appalling horrors. They have seen their homes destroyed, loved ones killed, been tortured or trafficked. They have taken long, terrifying journeys to reach safety."

****

Then we see an article in the *Guardian* just today (30th October, 2023) by Amelia Gentleman who exposes the dreadful treatment of refugee children and quotes from interviews with seven young asylum seekers in Yorkshire this week. Ms. Gentleman is an award winning journalist, winning the Paul Foot Award, the Cudlipp Award, an Amnesty Award, and many others.

So many times the Border Force together with the Home Office tries to classify the children as adults and they use every possible means they can to achieve this. The Refugee Council has warned of the dangers of this and has also warned of the risk of then forcing them to share rooms with adults.

The young refugees who were interviewed all said they told border guards that they were 16 or 17 on arrival in the UK by small boat in August and September – but all said they were wrongly classified as adults by officials and given ages between 22 and 26.

Refugee Council staff who subsequently interviewed them, and verified the identity documents of those who have them, verified these documents and accused the authorities of making mistakes. Or, as I would put it, deliberately changing the evidence.

One boy from Eritrea said *"Maybe the interpreter gave them the wrong information. They made me 10 years older; I couldn't understand it,"* He is uncomfortable in the adult hotel and said he has felt suicidal. *"I'm sharing with a man who's about 30. I feel lost. Sometimes I put my head under the bedding and cry. I miss my mum."*

Another boy whose identity papers show he is 16, was classified at the border as 22. *"They put my birthday down correctly, but they put 2001 instead of 2007. I said: 'That's not the right year,' and they said, 'Don't worry, a case worker will sort it out for you later.'"* He was unable to rectify the mistake and has been put in a hotel room with a 40-year-old man, who smokes out of the window, attracting trouble from the hotel security guards.

The Home Office says it wants to stop adult applicants "posing as children as a way of accessing support they are not entitled to", but charities say asylum seekers have little awareness of what support might be available.

Of course they don't know anything at all about that sort of detail or any detail come to that. They are just terrified young people asking for sanctuary.

All the children interviewed said they didn't feel safe.

****

So many of them also appear to be being housed in **adult prisons** which hold significant numbers of sex offenders.

According to the most recent inspection of Elmley prison, the block where foreign nationals are held and which also houses sex offenders, of 14 unaccompanied children so far identified by staff at 'Humans For Rights Network' as being sent to an adult prison, one is believed to have been 14 when they spent seven months in Elmley.

Most of the cases involve Sudanese or South Sudanese children who travelled to the UK via Libya, with most appearing to have been trafficked or having experienced some form of exploitation.

Maddie Harris, of 'Human Rights Network' said: "The children are always deeply harmed by the time they have spent in prison in the UK, expressing clearly how they are unable to sleep, do not understand why they were held there and struggle to speak about their time there."

She added: "It should be made clear that neither adult nor child should be criminalised for arriving in the UK to claim asylum, an offence that clearly contravenes the refugee convention."

Ms. Harris referred to a recent court ruling that unaccompanied minors should be looked after by councils "where they can be kept safe and recover."

And in recent written questions, the Home Office has refused to answer a question about how many **unaccompanied children are currently in hotel accommodation**. They have also refused to provide information on how many unaccompanied children they have detained for more than 24 hours which is the legal limit.

However I understand that the government had promised local authorities that asylum seekers who had been classified as adults but who claimed that they were children would **not** be sent to RAF Wethersfield in Essex which has been converted to Home Office Accommodation.

And then I read that actually this is what they have just done. So they are in breach of their own rules. *(Molly Blackall of* the i*)*

****

And the United Nations in Geneva on 11th April 2023 stated that: – "The United Kingdom must ensure the protection of all children seeking asylum without discrimination and put an end to the practice of placing unaccompanied children in hotels. We are deeply concerned at reports that unaccompanied asylum-seeking children are going missing and are at high risk of being trafficked within the UK," the UN experts said.

They expressed alarm at the current policy and practice of housing unaccompanied asylum-seeking children in temporary hotel accommodations instead of under the responsibility of local authorities.

"The current policy of placing unaccompanied asylum-seeking children in hotels places them outside of the UK child protection system and is discriminatory", the expert said, adding that failures and gaps in child protection heighten risks of trafficking.

They stressed the urgent need to trace the missing children, and to provide human rights compliant reception conditions and protection for unaccompanied children seeking asylum – without discrimination on grounds of nationality, migration status, race, ethnicity and/or gender.

"The UK Government appears to be failing to abide by its core obligations under international human rights law to ensure the best interests of the child, without discrimination, and to prevent trafficking of children," they said.

They noted reports that 4,600 unaccompanied children have been housed in six hotels since June 2021, and that 440 of these children had disappeared and 220 remained unaccounted for as of 23 January 2023, the majority of whom were Albanian nationals.

"The practice has allegedly developed in a climate of increasing hostility towards victims of trafficking and contemporary forms of slavery, refugees, asylum seekers and migrants," they said. Some Members of Parliament have reportedly been critical of victims of trafficking seeking protection under the Modern Slavery Act and the National Referral Mechanism, undermining the State's obligation to protect victims and to prevent trafficking and contemporary forms of slavery. The experts have been in contact with the UK Government regarding their serious concerns."

So absolute criticism of this Conservative government's treatment of refugee children from the United Nations.

And here are some more facts from The Refugee Council.

In the last 12 months 79% of claims by children which were actually assessed were granted asylum or another form of leave to remain.

A further 93 unaccompanied children were granted short-term leave to remain which lasts for two and a half years only.

The top country of origin for claims for asylum from children is Afghanistan.

As they say "war and persecution often divides refugees from their families but there are few straightforward legal ways for refugees to safely join loved ones in Britain."

In the UK there is something called a refugee family reunion visa. Well I was certainly not aware of this. But before you get carried away with the humanity of this you need to be aware that they are "incredibly restrictive."

For some inane reason current UK law allows adult refugees rebuilding their lives in the country to sponsor their immediate family members to join them, but unaccompanied child refugees are completely deprived of this right.

****

You might have read about the instance when Robert Jenrick, Immigration Minister, ordered some murals of Disney characters at a children's asylum centre in Kent to be painted over.

He said it was a law enforcement centre not a welcoming committee. I wrote about this on page 446 of my book "**Britain Betrayed**" on the 3rd July 2023 and I and many others could not believe the sheer nastiness of this approach. It later emerged that a child-friendly mural at a separate detention camp had also been painted over at a cost to the tax payer of £1,549.52.

It was all over Twitter and many, many people including cartoonists and artists and young children in primary schools offered to repaint it or to make colouring books. The explosion of kindness was heart-warming.

Guy Venables, a cartoonist and member of the PCO, (Professional Cartoonists Organisation) said his response was "one of pure rage, white anger".

He and other cartoonists discussed "a well-aimed, calm but wholly positive response". The idea of a colouring book introducing British culture to newly arrived children was perfect, he said, and requests went out to the nation's cartoonists.

Well today (20th November) I hear that this colouring book has been officially launched this week. Supporters were told that £3 was needed to fund each book plus colouring pencils. More than enough money for an initial run of 1,000 books was raised overnight. The printing costs were crowd-funded by '38 Degrees' and it is already being used by young children in asylum centres. Every single cartoonist approached said yes and some of the top names are there. Contributors include Quentin Blake, Ralph Steadman, Chris Riddell, Ros Asquith, Nicola Jennings and Terry Gilliam.

Guy Venables said that each child will be handed "something very normal, a colouring book. Just a book. Maybe one day they will discover that they had the attention of a whole nation's cartoonists who stood in solidarity on their side, who were inspired to collectively shine a light into the dark and show them that somebody cared."

They are now planning a second book. Matthew McGregor, chief executive of '38 Degrees' said "The British public who chipped in to fund the colouring book are sending a clear message to the government: give children arriving in this country, having fled war and persecution, the warm welcome to Britain they deserve." So listen carefully Mr. Jenrick. When you and your colleagues such as Suella Braverman say that you speak for the British public you are actually so out of step that you could be on the other side of the moon. You lie. You obviously have no idea what the general public think.

All these wonderful people restore my faith in humanity.

****

When I was a volunteer speaker for the charity 'Save the Children' one of my talks was called '**What it is like to be a refugee child?**'. I always started by quoting their founder Eglantyne Jebb when she said that "All war, whether just or unjust, victorious or disastrous, is waged against the child." All wars produce refugees and nearly half of all refugees are children. We heard so many stories from refugee children all of them heart breaking. These are some of their voices.

"Suddenly having a life that is often more difficult than the one you grew up with is really hard. Becoming a refugee or simply running away from war is a little war of its own."

"If you are a refugee some part of your life is always missing and that is your home."

"I miss my family so much. They are all over Europe and I know that the only place I will ever see my family and friends is back on my village."

"We are not here because we are seeking a better life. We are here because we are seeking a safe environment."

"We don't want to be refugees. We want to be building up our own countries and wanting them to be good places in which to live."

"We are not refugees by choice. We are refugees by situation and circumstance."

And I used to end my talks by saying that Britain has a long history of offering refuge to those who need it. And indeed we did.

But not now. Not any-more.

****

"Give me your tired, your poor,
Your huddled masses
Yearning to breathe free..."

Emma Lazarus, 'The New Colossus'

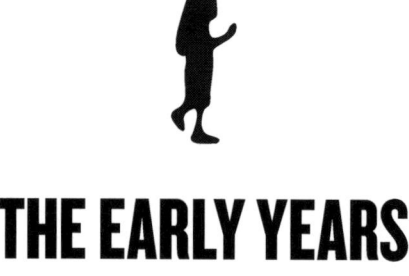

THE EARLY YEARS

The first seven years of a child's life are universally acknowledged to be the most important in their social, physical, emotional, and cognitive development. Indeed as the great Greek philosopher Aristotle once said, "Give me a child until he is 7 and I will show you the man."

This is repeated by eminent people and organsations until you think it must be accepted by every government.

Ofsted said on the GOV.UK web site on the 8th September 2023 "that frequent interactions between children and adults are fundamental to developing all young children's knowledge in the prime areas of learning – communication and language, physical development and personal, social and emotional development (PSED). Every interaction between a practitioner and a child plays an important role in building the knowledge and skills children will need."

Amanda Spielman, His Majesty's Chief Inspector, said: "A strong foundation in the early years is crucial for children's success throughout their education and beyond. The research clearly shows that early years practitioners who focus on the prime areas, and understand that every interaction is a teaching opportunity, leave children equipped with the tools they need to thrive."

The Princess of Wales launched 'Shaping Us' campaign to boost understanding of early childhood's formative role and said "it is more important than ever" to support the development of young children" as she launches this early years campaign. "The way we develop, through our experiences, relationships and surroundings during our early childhood fundamentally shapes our whole lives.

"It affects everything from our ability to form relationships and thrive at work, to our mental and physical wellbeing as adults and the way we parent our own children.

"These are the most preventive years. By focusing our collective time, energy and resources to build a supportive, nurturing world around the youngest members of our society and those caring for them, we can make a huge difference to the health and happiness of generations to come."

The 'Shaping Us' campaign aims to improve society's understanding of the importance of early childhood in shaping adulthood and society as a whole.

The long-term project, launched on Wednesday 15th November 2023 by the 'Royal Foundation Centre for Early Childhood,' is said to be Catherine's "life's work", which she hopes will influence attitudes towards children in the early-years period of their lives. "All of society has a role to play in this, even if you are not directly involved in a child's life, because we are all responsible for building a more compassionate world in which our children can grow, learn and live.

"In these difficult times, it is more important than ever to help support parents and caregivers provide loving safe and secure homes for their babies and young children to survive."

****

And then there is the 'NSPCC' which does a huge amount for the most vulnerable children in our society.

They say that "Early help and early intervention services can be provided at any stage in a child or young person's life, from the early years right through to adolescence. Services can be delivered to parents, children, or whole families.

"Providing timely support is vital. Identifying and addressing a child or family's needs early on can increase protective factors that positively influence a child's wellbeing, and decrease risk factors that may be impacting a child's life negatively."

Research suggests that early help and intervention can:

- protect children from harm
- reduce the need for a referral to child protection services
- improve children's long-term outcomes
- improve children's home and family life
- support children to develop strengths and skills to prepare them for adult life.

Some groups of children may be more likely to need early help than their peers. These include children who:

- have special educational needs
- are disabled
- are young carers
- display disruptive or anti-social behaviour
- experience difficulties at home, such as domestic abuse, parental substance abuse or parental mental health problems
- are involved in, or at risk of, offending
- are in care, leaving care or preparing to leave care
- have poor attendance at, or are excluded from, school
- are young parents (or about to become young parents)
- are experiencing housing issues
- misuse drugs or alcohol
- are being bullied or bullying others
- have poor general health
- have mental health issues

****

We also had the 'Sure Start' programme which was created and developed under New Labour as a way of improving the educational and life chances of socially and economically disadvantaged children. These centres offered families access to services including childcare, healthcare, parenting classes, job skills and playgroups.

They were brilliant and on 16 Aug 2021 Pippa Crerar, when political editor in the *Mirror*, wrote that:

"More than 13,000 hospital admissions of children a year were prevented by Sure Start."

"The 'Institute for Fiscal Studies' found that the benefits of the centres were 'substantial' with children in poorer neighbourhoods getting most out of them."

"The IFS research, funded by the' Nuffield Foundation', found that the early years programme delivered long-lasting health benefits for children well into their teenage years".

"Sure Start centres, which brought together health, parenting support and childcare for the under-5s, received £1.8bn a year at their 2009 peak."

****

So what has happened?

Well what has happened is that child-care in the early years has been demoted, defunded, deprioritised, and thoroughly neglected by Conservative governments.

In 2018 **Patrick Butler,** the *Guardian Social policy editor* wrote that:

"By 2010, there were 3,600 centres in the UK. Before that year's general election, the Conservative leader at the time, David Cameron, promised to protect funding for 'Sure Start', but this pledge quickly evaporated amid swingeing cuts to local authority budgets.

Over the next seven years, early years' provision bore the brunt of cuts to children's services."

And it just went on from there.

According to the 'Sutton Trust', over 500 centres were closed during the following years and they said that "most councils have had to abandon the original 'Sure Start' ideal of an open-access, neighbourhood-based facility for parents and preschool children, adding: "Services are now 'hollowed out'."

Sir Peter Lampl, founder of the 'Sutton Trust', said: "Good-quality early years provision makes a substantial difference in the development of children, especially those who come from the poorest homes. It is a serious issue that the services that 'Sure Start' centres offer are much more thinly spread than they were a decade ago."

Spending has fallen by more than two –thirds over the last decade under the Tories.

Charities say cuts to public services mean many are not seen by a health visitor at two and a half as they should be, and the closure of children's centres has resulted in struggling families falling beneath the radar.

And today we hear horrific stories about young children who are still suffering from the after effects of the pandemic.

I am really grateful to Anne Fazackerley who highlighted these concerns in an article for the *Observer* on 7th October this year, 2023.

Children are just not prepared to start school and she says that in some deprived areas children are arriving at school not yet potty-trained and many are arriving at school in push chairs.

It is crucial that all children are seen and assessed by a health visitor during their first five years but the NSPCC has found that 38% of families are not receiving their mandated antenatal health visit, and a quarter are missing their contact when their child turns one.

NSPCC head of policy and public affairs, Almudena Lara, said: "At present, England offers a limited service in comparison to Scotland, which offers 11 mandatory visits, Wales that offers nine and Northern Ireland with seven."

Apparently only 1 in 10 parents with children under two saw a health visitor face-to-face during the pandemic..

Jane Harris, chief executive of the charity 'Speech and Language UK,' which published research in September showing that 1.9 million children are behind with talking and understanding words, said that insufficient health visitors meant "loads of children aren't being seen at two and a half years old as they should be".

More than half of teachers have told the charity they don't know how to help children with speech and language difficulties, and Harris says schools that are struggling to recruit and retain teaching assistants because of low pay often don't have enough staff to give extra support.

Anne Longfield, the government's former Children's Commissioner, who now chairs the independent 'Commission on Young Lives', told the *Observer* that many children starting school have speech and language delays because they have had dummies in their mouths for so long over the pandemic and since. She said "that a lack of early support for struggling families, combined with undiagnosed special educational needs, has caused an 'outbreak' of very young children who can't cope in a classroom environment."

And this is the other shocking statistic. Ms. Longfield says "Children as young as four are being excluded from schools in England in increasing numbers as they struggle to cope in a classroom setting, with many still in nappies or unable to talk fully.

According to the latest government data, 11,695 children aged five and under were given fixed-term exclusions in England in the 2021-22 academic year, which was 11% higher than 2018-19."

This is unbelievable and an indictment on way this government simply doesn't care for our children.

As Ms. Longfield continues, **"Anyone who discovers that children of four, five and six are being excluded is in utter shock. It just feels so wrong."**

It feels absolutely terrible.

She described meeting a group of parents in north London whose children had been excluded in the first few years of primary school. "One five-year-old child had been excluded 17 times between Easter and Christmas. The child was then sent to a pupil referral unit where there were no other young children and they had to be put in a room by themselves," she explained.

This is sheer cruelty to children. There is no other word.

****

So we waited for the March budget with baited breath to see how the Chancellor would help.

Well they have tried to replace the excellent 'Sure Start' programmes with an Education Hub as they slowly came to realise that closing so many 'Sure Start' centres was a dreadful idea.

I read this on the Education Hub GOV.UK website.

*From **April 2024**, working parents of two-year-olds will be able to access 15 hours of free childcare.*

*From **September 2024**, 15 hours of free childcare will be extended to all children from the age of nine months.*

*From **September 2025**, working parents of children under the age of five will be entitled to 30 hours free childcare per week.*

This staggered approach will give childcare providers time to prepare for the changes, ensuring there are enough providers ready to meet demand.

*From **September 2023**, one member of staff will be allowed to look after five children, up from four children which is the current rule.*

But before we all say well that sounds brilliant I see a report by Michael Savage of the *Guardian* on 19th March which explains it all and the first paragraph gives us all a sense of foreboding.

"An eye-catching pledge for a huge expansion of free childcare provision was a main giveaway in the chancellor's budget last week," he writes. "However, while childcare providers have welcomed extra help for parents, nurseries across England, speaking to the *Observer*, said that the plan risked having a "catastrophic" impact on the sector without an overhauling of central funding."

This is one of the problems with this government. They love announcing new money for this and that but always forget about the workers and the people needed to staff everything. (Remember the Nightingale hospitals?)

Mr. Savage goes on to say that "The budget plan will see 30 hours a week of free childcare given to all children aged from nine months to four years, though its introduction will be staggered. At present, parents of three and four-year-olds can claim 15 or 30 hours of free childcare, depending on their circumstances.

Hunt promised an increase of free hours funding of £204m from this September, eventually rising to £288m next year. However, it is well below independent estimates of the costs nurseries face and full funding details have not been revealed."

He goes on to quote the people who actually know the system and who are on the front line of the child-care programmes.

"This will be the end of nurseries," said **Mel Hart, owner of Albion House nursery and the Old School nursery in Grantham, Lincolnshire.** "We are already underfunded by approximately £2.50 per hour, per child for the three and four-year-olds. Over 5,000 nurseries are said to have closed in the last year. If more are struggling financially, more will also close. Then there will be nowhere for children to go so that parents can go to work."

Olivia Foley of the Hungry Caterpillar nurseries, most of which are in London, said it was already difficult to fill vacancies, as the work was hard and wages already higher elsewhere – even before any further spending squeeze.

"We have got so many vacancies; we've got nurseries where we're holding registration down to around 60% because we just can't get the staff," she said. "The idea that we're going to be able to provide all these additional places – unless there's a workforce development plan there just won't be the staff to deliver it."

Caroline Nutting of the Little Acorns preschool in Leigh-on-Sea, Essex, said: "We would have to make redundancies, have less staff and the care and high standard provision would end up being affected."

Sarah Jacomb, owner of the Toybox day nursery in East Grinstead, West Sussex, said the idea of free hours was "simply not true and very misleading". She backed helping parents, but added: "Parents are now expecting free childcare and are oblivious to the fact that nurseries will have to somehow bridge the gap between what the government will pay them and what it actually costs them."

Neil Leitch, head of education charity the Early Years Alliance, said: "The levels of funding and the 30-hour expansion plans announced in the budget show the government has underestimated just how serious the issues facing the early years' sector are. We urge the Treasury to engage in discussions with us so, together, we can work out how these plans will work in practice."

Well now that would be a good idea. But do you really mean to tell me that the Chancellor did not consult you before the budget? It is, all of it, beyond belief.

****

Well, if you think as I do, that that was all beyond belief just read this.

I have already written about the government trying to prevent senior educators from speaking at conferences if they have been found to be criticising the government's education policies on social media and here are some more..

It would appear that they have been looking at the social media accounts of teachers and teaching assistants and they are actually keeping files on anyone who criticises their education policy. People are now being threatened with the with-holding of funding if they talk at particular events.

I am once again indebted to the brilliant journalist Anne Fazackerley of *the Observer*.

On the 21st October 2023 she writes that "Dr. Mine Conkbayir, an award-winning early-childhood author and consultant, was told by the organisers of an early-years conference for nursery staff and childminders in Bristol in March, for which she was due to give the keynote speech that the DfE had threatened to withdraw funding for the conference if she spoke. They were unhappy about her criticisms of their policies on social media."

She told the *Observer*: "I felt like I had been punched in the stomach. I was frightened. I thought, 'They are trying to silence me and they have so much power.'"

Eventually she was given permission to speak but only when the department for education had checked her speech beforehand.

Others were told they could only speak on Zoom in order presumably so that officials could "cut us off if they didn't like what we were saying."

In the end they felt they had no choice but to pull out of the talks. A key speaker, Julie Harmieson, director of education and strategy at training organisation 'Trauma Informed Schools', pulled out in solidarity. In an email to the organisers, she said: "I would not feel comfortable speaking, knowing that Mine has been silenced in the way she has."

Dr. Conkbayir, like other early-years experts, disagreed with the recommendation of putting very small children who misbehaved in "time out" or taking away their toys as a punishment – strategies she believes are psychologically harmful as well as unlikely to work.

She added: "The more they try to silence me, the louder I will get. Everyone in the sector is so scared of the DfE and Ofsted, but we have to question things or the people who will suffer are the children."

Everyone has a duty to shout out against what they perceive to be harmful practices against anyone but especially against children.

And then we hear the usual weasel words from the government.

Asked whether they were monitoring the social media of teaching staff, the DfE said it would not be appropriate to comment on individual cases and that it was standard practice to carry out due diligence before engaging external experts.

Big Brother is alive and well.

****

New Ofsted figures published this June (2023) show a major drop in the number of childcare places since March 2022.

Commenting on these latest figures from Ofsted, Jonathan Broadbery, director of policy and communications at National Day Nurseries Association (NDNA) said it "has to be a wake-up call for the Government. Nearly 5,000 fewer providers, 400 nurseries lost and 24,500 fewer places for children, all at a time when providers need to be gearing up to offer more funded places from April".

Purmina Tanuku |OBE, Chief Executive of NDNA said "The alarming rate at which nurseries are continuing to close puts in doubt the government's ability to deliver on their promise of more funded child-care from April 2024".

She sad that "From April the average nursery's wage bill will shoot up by 14% – and yet they are only increasing their fees to parents by around 8% or lower in areas of deprivation in an effort to keep places affordable. Some parents just can't pay more and those nurseries will struggle to keep going.

"We were shocked to find that 83% of nurseries do not expect to make any surplus at all and 38% are operating at a loss – this increases to 45% in the 20% most deprived areas."

Neil Leitch, chief executive of the 'Early Years Alliance', said: "Years of underfunding and completely disregarding the sector time have left us with a shell of an early years sector with provider numbers plummeting at an alarming rate."

So nurseries continue to close and UK child-care costs continues to be the third highest in Europe behind Slovakia and Switzerland

****

And today (5th November) we hear that one in five mothers of young children have considered giving up their careers due to the difficulties of balancing child-care and work. Jemima Olchawski the chief executive of the 'Fawcett Society' said "employers should "end the motherhood penalty" and support flexible working and more affordable child-care.

The chief executive of 'Totaljobs' talking about mothers said that "businesses need to create an environment where they can flourish. With critical labour shortages the pressures of children could ultimately have a longer-term impact on our ever-shrinking workforce."

This is very true and requires some serious joined–up thinking. Who is going to do that do you think?

Meanwhile child-care continues to be expensive and unaffordable for many. Nurseries struggle to make ends meet, children are shuttled from one place to another, and the government looks the other way.

****

But then I see something which gives me hope.

Whilst researching this book I come across so many interesting places and charities and amazing people that I otherwise would not have heard about.

This is one such place. It is called the **Liverpool Hope University** and this is how it describes itself on the web site.

"It is distinctive in that it is the only university foundation in Europe (and the USA) where Catholic and Anglican colleges have come together to form an integrated, ecumenical, Christian foundation. It has happened in Liverpool and nowhere else in Europe largely because of the presence in the 1980s of two remarkable church leaders: Bishop David Sheppard, the Bishop of the Anglican Diocese, and Archbishop Derek Worlock, the Archbishop of the Catholic Archdiocese that extends from Liverpool across the north of England. They confessed their faith to each other and took their congregations to visit each other's cathedrals, a symbolic act of Christians working together in the context of northern Irish religious sectarianism.

"When the three colleges (St Katharine's 1844, Notre Dame College 1856 and Christ's College 1964) came together the name 'Hope' came from Hope Street that links both cathedrals - a real example of what can happen when people unite and work together for the common good.

"In 2019 we celebrated 175 years since the founding of our first college in 1844; in that year there were only six universities in England (two of them medieval) but none of them admitted women, Catholics or Jews. **The founding colleges of Liverpool Hope University were among the first few institutions to begin opening up higher education to the vast majority of England's population."**

Well I say "wow" to that and am amazed that I haven't heard of it before. But of course many will remember those two wonderful theologians, David Sheppard and Derek Worlock.

And also at Liverpool Hope University, its well-established **early years' education courses** are about more than education. As Prof Cate Carroll-Meehan, dean and head of the school of education, says: "When you think about how a child develops into an adult, it really is those first five years which are critical in terms of not just physical development and emotional development, but how they regulate their emotions, how they learn to get on with other people, and the values they form – their attitudes and prejudices."

And this is amazing: Based on the belief that working with young children requires an understanding of pedagogy, psychology, sociology and philosophy, one of Liverpool Hope's new qualifications is a BA in early childhood studies with graduate practitioner competencies. It requires students to complete 80 days in a range of placements – such as children's centres, schools, hospitals, wellbeing and family support services – alongside their degree. The first cohort graduated this year. "They are entering the profession well-versed in child development and pedagogy but also in policy and advocacy," says Dr. Clionagh Boyle, the university's head of early childhood. "And they will need those skills if we are serious about bringing real change for and with children."

This is a wonderful new degree for teachers of young children.

They talk about the excellence of the 'Sure Start' programme which was the flagship Labour policy, announced in 1998 in Parliament and also of the wonderful programme introduced by Labour on 2003 called '**Every Child Matters**.' This was introduced to move on a bit from the 'Sure Start' programmes which were causing some concern because of the variability of local 'Sure Start' service provision and about the programme's ability to reach the poorest families, identified by early evaluation work. This strengthened the case for universalising the service.

" 'Sure Start' is a good example of a policy that could really have made a difference long-term but was decimated under the austerity policy of subsequent governments," says Dr Boyle, "The lip service that is paid to the importance of young children while electioneering doesn't translate to policy that addresses child poverty," she says.

Yes indeed we all know that. But what a marvellous programme for anyone wanting to make a difference to the lives of our children by teaching in the early years.

And how great that I can finish a chapter with such an up-lifting account.

******

"A child must know that he is a miracle,
that since the beginning of the world
there hasn't been, and until the end of
the world there will not be,
another child like him"

Pablo Casals (Spanish Cellist)

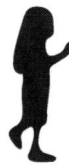

WHAT OF THE FUTURE?

People often ask me the questions "Well would the other lot be any better?" and "Aren't they all as bad as each other?"

Having done a lot of research I can honestly say that absolutely yes they will be better and absolutely they are quite different from this present lot.

First I need to talk about **Sir Keir Starmer**, leader of the Opposition. He gets a lot of criticism for not being 'charismatic' enough, nor exciting enough.

To which I reply 'I'm done with charisma and excitability thank you.'

As we hear extracts from the Covid inquiry we learn about the complete chaotic shambles that existed in No 10 during the pandemic under the premiership of Boris Johnson. It was a disgrace.

In Keir Starmer we have someone who is serious, calm, and intelligent, with an analytical mind, an attention to detail and a huge degree of gravitas. He has also put in place an excellent shadow cabinet. Wes Streeting, Yvette Cooper, Bridget Phillipson, Rachel Reeves, David Lammy, Angela Rayner, Thangam Debbonaire, Anneliese Dodds, Lisa Nandy, John Healey, **Jonathan Ashworth** and others are all grown-ups, brimming with ideas as to how to improve the lives of the people in this country and especially the lives of our children. So let us take a closer look at what they are proposing.

Bridget Phillipson is the Shadow Education Secretary so I will begin with her.

She certainly understands the importance of the early years, as in July she told the *Guardian* that, "We need to raise the standing of the [early years] sector, make it part of the education system so that it is regarded with the same parity as our schools,"

"What you achieve in the early years makes such a big difference."

And as part of its national excellence programme Labour has vowed to recruit 6,500 new teachers.

In a speech earlier this year Bridget Phillipson said "The priority for any secretary of state for education has to be making sure that children can go to schools that are fit for purpose. But the challenge is more than that. It is to break down the barriers."

Her vision seems to be to transform state schools into places that children want to attend, and are proud to do so, in which teachers want to teach, and in which parents have confidence and place their trust. "Places that are central to the community," she adds.

She is worried about absenteeism among pupils, levels of which are higher in areas of the north of England, where GCSE and A-level results are less good. There is a clear connection. "We need children back in school. We are seeing a real problem with absenteeism."

And in her **Conference speech** she said that one big idea that is now firm policy is to bring in breakfast clubs for all pupils in all primary schools in England, as a priority and in a first Labour term. It will cost £365m a year, ensuring that children from poorer backgrounds can start the school day with a good meal.

"It is also that they will get a softer start to the day, time with their friends," she said. "It will be of educational benefit too, helping concentration and the ability to learn. Under an inevitably cash-strapped Labour government, money will be found to pay for more teachers by ending tax breaks for private schools, a policy the Institute for Fiscal Studies says will raise about £1.6bn a year."

The charity 'Magic Breakfast' welcomed the announcement "that a Labour Government will introduce fully funded breakfast clubs for every primary school in England."

Problems with retention of teaching staff will be addressed by promising extra payments of £2,400 to those in the very early stages of their careers in England to try to stop them leaving.

This is such a big contrast to Gillian Keegan's speech to the Conservative Party Conference. The first five minutes were entirely devoted to her and her background and to how well she has done. She then told the Conservative lie when she said that **"our phonics checks are ensuring children leave school able to read properly."**

This is a blatant lie because we hear Amanda Spielman, Her Majesty's Chief Inspector, writing about the importance of reading – **and the need to help struggling readers as they start secondary school.**

"I am worried about children who are still struggling to read when they start secondary school." she says.

"Children are tested in the last year of primary school, known as SATs. This year's tests showed that nearly 175,000 pupils did not meet the expected standard in reading. That means around a quarter of all Year 7s still have a reading age of below 11."

We all know the importance of reading because without that there is nothing else.

So why is this the situation then?

We know about work done by 'The National Literacy Trust' to try to get designated reading spaces and libraries into schools. Why does the government keep perpetuating these lies instead of trying to solve the problem of a lack of libraries in schools?

And here is another amazing charity.

I discovered the 'West London Zone' charity when working on my previous books and I was blown away by the work they were doing.

This is now they describe their work on their website.

"West London Zone is a collective impact initiative supporting young people in West London – a three-square mile area around Harrow Road in London. This area is home to around 66,000 young people aged 0 to 25. The Zone is deeply divided by wealth and life chances; it has some of the most prosperous neighbourhoods in the country, but also some of the most deprived areas.

West London Zone found that 20% of the children in the area exhibited risk factors such as social exclusion, educational disadvantage, and poor mental well-being that could prevent them from living a happy and independent life if left unaddressed."

They then describe what they do.

This is their solution.

"Together with their community, WLZ designed a **Collective Impact** approach to leverage the local "social assets" – such as charities, nurseries, schools, statutory services, and other community groups – around a shared vision. As the 'backbone' for this initiative, WLZ actively supports each partner and provides a Link Worker for each child, who builds a trusted, lasting relationship with the child and their family, helping them set their own goals for the future and working with charity partners on the ground to ensure that delivery is consistent and tailored to each individual. The support programme for each child lasts for 2 years.

In December 2017, the WLZ programme was extended to cover areas of deprivation in Kensington and Chelsea."

Well this brilliant charity went to the Labour Party Conference and was able to speak to Bridget Phillipson's team, Josh McAllister, Executive Chair of 'What Works Centre for Children & Families' and Anne Longfield, Chair of the 'Commission on Young Lives', and also Dame Rachel de Souza, who described West London Zone as providing a bridge for schools into community assets and opportunities.

Their CEO, Louisa Mitchell, also spoke on a panel event hosted by 'Onward UK' alongside the Greater Manchester Mayor, Andy Burnham, and representatives from the 'Sutton Trust' and 'Ambition Institute'. The panel discussed the role of schools, the importance of a whole-child approach and the need to harness the whole system around children and their families.

In fact this approach was central to the whole debate. They said, "It was encouraging that one of the main areas of consensus was the need for a whole-child, whole system approach for support which aligns closely with our programme. Crucially there was also an appetite to better connect schools, children and families with wider assets across the community, which echoes a key element of our Link Work model."

Andy Burnham discussed the fragmented nature of the current system and the need for greater connectivity between schools and services across the local community. He was keen to stress that the issues faced by young people in his region are similar to the challenges Louisa described in West London. They said, "it was encouraging to hear him express his support for the West London Zone model."

They are now in liaison with his office to arrange a follow-up meeting to discuss their shared priorities and opportunities for future joint working.

Altogether they were delighted to hear Bridget Phillipson speaking about the importance of both early intervention and the need to design solutions with the local communities – both of which are core principles of the WLZ model.

So this was a very useful visit to the Labour Conference and as they say "One of the main areas of consensus across events and speakers was the need for a whole-child, whole system approach for support. This is a fundamental element of our model, and it was positive to hear such widespread support for this approach."

NEXT STEPS

"The WLZ team are now working towards arranging follow-up meetings with the key stakeholders we engaged with at the Labour conference, including Andy Burnham and the Labour Education team. We look forward to sharing further updates on our public affairs work in the coming months as the country prepares for the upcoming General Election."

Indeed this all sounds a very positive future for our children's education. I think we can see which government **does** act and **does** care and **has** plans to put into action some excellent children's programmes.

****

Then we look at **Wes Streeting and what he envisages for the NHS as shadow secretary of State for Health and Social Care.**

We hear him talking at conference on the 11th October 2023.

He says that "Children in Britain should be part of the healthiest generation ever." Well I think we are a long way from that at the moment.

But he is realistic when he goes on to say that: "I'm blunt about the fact that the NHS is no longer the envy of the world, not to undermine it, but to reassure people that we've noticed. I argue that our NHS must modernise or die, not as a threat but a choice. The crisis really is that existential."

This is good because I say over and over again that if you don't acknowledge a problem then you cannot fix it. And this government's answer to every criticism is "We are chucking loads of money into it" or words to that effect but they never admit there is a problem.

After saying Labour's reform agenda will "turn the NHS on its head", Mr. Streeting added: "A neighbourhood health service as much as a National Health Service, pioneering cutting-edge treatment and technology, preventing ill-health, not just treating it."

Then he talks about schools and how important it is to look after our children.

"The better Britain which the next Labour government will build, will come not from obsessing about structures, but from a fresh focus; a focus that draws on a ban on junk food adverts targeted at children, action against vaping companies pushing nicotine products on youngsters, breakfast clubs at every primary school and supervised tooth-brushing in schools."

Then he goes on to talk about the crisis in dentistry. I read some dreadful facts about tooth decay in children.

'Full Facts Fact check' says that for children aged one to 17 the top two causes of hospital admission in 2022/23 were viral infection and acute tonsillitis, then tooth decay. Based on the individual age groups provided in the data, the five to nine-year-olds age group was the only one where tooth decay was the most common reason for being admitted to hospital. This is confirmed by the Local Government Association.

Every day, 160 children and teenagers in England have tooth extractions while under general anaesthetic in hospital, according to the LGA.

The British Dental Association has commented that these hospital admissions could be avoided as tooth decay is entirely preventable.

"The government must take urgent action to address this dental crisis, including tackling staff shortages, increasing health education and reforming the broken system that has driven dentists away from offering NHS appointments," they say.

So that's why Wes Streeting says that Labour has pledged to provide an extra 700,000 urgent dentist appointments and reform the NHS dental contract, as part of a package of measures to rescue NHS dentistry.

Of course nothing can be achieved over-night and it will be a long journey but they are recognising the problem and they have a plan.

Then we hear what Wes Streeting plans for the distressing stories we are hearing about young mothers being forced to **steal baby formula milk** as baby banks run out of supplies.

Metro has started a fantastic campaign which calls for the government to scrap guidelines surrounding how infant formula can be bought. It is the case that while customers can use loyalty points and store gift vouchers to purchase the likes of alcohol, pet food and energy drinks, baby formula cannot be bought this way, however desperately it is needed.

It's an issue currently being highlighted by *Metro*'s 'Formula for Change' campaign in partnership with the family support charity 'Feed', which demands that the government gives the green light so cash-strapped families can afford to feed their families.

Backing this initiative, Wes Streeting told *Metro:* 'All families should be able to feed their babies and it's too hard for so many to afford to do so in this cost of living crisis.

"Regulations that prevent families from using foodbank vouchers to buy infant formula are no longer fit for purpose.

"We will not stand by while outdated restrictions have a damaging impact on those struggling to make ends meet, which is why Labour is backing The *Metro*'s 'Formula For Change' campaign.

"With Labour, retailers will be able to accept loyalty cards and vouchers as payment for infant formula to help families feed their children.

"We will urgently review existing legislation on infant formula, ensuring that regulation is protecting families and their babies, not making life more difficult for them.'

So that is a positive decision by Labour.

The cost of baby formula, also called infant formula or formula milk, has soared amid the deepening cost-of-living crisis. The cheapest brand has shot up by 45% in the past two years, 'First Steps Nutrition' previously found.

But we do hear that in response to the growing crisis, *Metro* teamed up with the charity 'Feed' to call on Rishi Sunak's government to urgently review their infant formula legislation. Has anything happened? As of the beginning of November 2023 no, nothing.

Meanwhile, supermarket chain 'Iceland' has also joined forces with *Metro* to support the campaign and **openly defied government policy** by slashing the price of its formula range by more than 20%.

Iceland's executive chairman Richard Walker, says 'bold action' from 'joint forces' is integral for any change.

He told *Metro.co.uk*: "I welcome the decision from the Labour Party to back the' Formula for Change' campaign. It is encouraging to know that under a future Labour government, Iceland's decision to accept loyalty points and vouchers as payment for formula milk wouldn't be breaking any guidelines.

"This shouldn't be about politics, or a debate between the merits of breastfeeding or using formula, this is about supporting the choices of UK parents as they navigate the cost of living crisis.

"It's about doing what is right, and supporting retailers like us so that we can do our part without facing consequences from archaic rules and regulations.

"In making this decision, Labour has demonstrated it is on the side of business, and ordinary families who are doing their best to get by every day."

There really are some wonderful people out there and the executive chairman of Iceland is one of them.

Kirston Robertson's full report in the *Metro* on the 30th October 2023 has highlighted the callousness of the government and the people who are refusing to accept this ruling and who are making a difference. Wes Streeting is on it.

And another excellent idea from him is to tackle the NHS's staffing crisis is **that newly qualified doctors and nurses in England could have their student loans written off**. Wow this would be wonderful.

Unions representing doctors and nurses welcomed Streeting's remarks. Prof Philip Banfield, the leader of the British Medical Association, said: "Student debt write-off could be an incentive to stay and, done properly, assist retention now. This is well worth exploring."

Nicola Ranger, the Royal College of Nursing's director of nursing, said: "Proposals from Labour in this area are constructive. Loans written off in exchange for service or the full removal of fees [for nursing degree courses] are options that must be on the table as part of making nursing attractive."

The 'Nuffield Trust' health think-tank has hailed student loans forgiveness as an example of the "bold policymaking" needed to address the NHS's workforce difficulties. It said the policy would reduce early career dropout, improve staff wellbeing and yield more applications for clinical courses.

Our children would have faster treatment and waiting lists would be brought down.

Wes Streeting is ready for action.

****

So we now look at the **shadow Home Secretary Yvette Cooper.**

Again we hear her speak at Conference.

A Labour government would set up a "tough love" youth programme to help combat crime, she said. It would be focused on tackling knife crime and a mental health crisis among young people.

"We need urgent interventions to stop young people getting drawn into crime or exploitation," she said.

She told the conference that knife crime had risen by 70% in eight years, adding "far too little is done" and a "generation is being failed".

Under cross-department proposals drawn up by Labour, a programme would be rolled out across the UK to identify vulnerable young people, with the aim of stopping them being pulled into lives of crime and violence.

The party has described the policy, which it says would cost £100m a year, as a "key part" of its mission to halve knife crime and youth violence within a decade.

It wants to create 90 youth hubs to bring together services for at-risk young people, modelled on the 'Sure Start' early-years initiative introduced by the Blair government.

And I never knew that it was actually Ms. Cooper who was one of the ministers responsible for launching 'Sure Start' in 1998. She got a huge ovation when talking about these at their conference.

Labour would place youth workers in A&E units, custody centres and pupil referral units to help those with mental health issues or straying into criminal behaviour.

For young people who repeatedly caused trouble in their community or were found to be carrying knives, "there also need to be stronger interventions and clear consequences to stop their behaviour escalating and to keep other young people safe", Ms. Cooper added.

Labour would "give young people their future back", she said.

Yes these are fine words and it won't be easy. But it is a good start.

****

But of course none of this will happen unless Labour produces a sound economy.

Rachel Reeves is the shadow Chancellor and prior to devoting her life to politics she spent her professional career as an **economist** working for the Bank of England, the British Embassy in Washington, and at Halifax Bank of Scotland. Her economic strategy has won plaudits from former Conservative chancellor Ken Clarke who called her "reassuring" and "responsible".

And also Mark Carney, who was hand-picked by former Tory chancellor George Osborne to be governor of the Bank of England, stunned the Labour conference with a video address saying: "**Rachel Reeves is a serious economist**. She began her career at the Bank of England, so she understands the big picture. But, crucially she understands the economics of work, of place and family. It is beyond time we put her energy and ideas into action."

Well you cannot get more genuine praise than that.

****

So these are some of the people in the shadow cabinet who will have the most influence on our children's lives. They are ready to govern. They have good plans in place. They care about the well-fare of our children. The comparison with those who have been in government for 13 years is stark.

I conclude by looking further at their leader.

Sir Keir Starmer is often accused of being boring but being Prime Minister is not supposed to be a cabaret act. He used to be the head of the Crown Prosecution Service. No he isn't particularly charismatic but if it is charisma that produced Boris Johnson's win then I do not want any more of it. For too long we have been ruled by the incompetent and the uncaring and the damage done to our children is, in many cases, irreparable. For that alone they will not be forgiven.

Sir Keir Starmer has said a lot about children's education and it is a really interesting mix.

Sir Keir will promise to break the "class ceiling" with a goal of half a million more children reaching their early learning targets by 2030 and with a target to recruit 6,500 more teachers into shortage subjects.

To help reach the 2030 target, the party will double the number of health visitors, provide further mental health support for parents, as well as early years speech and language therapy - which would be funded by scrapping the VAT exemption on private schools.

Well the private schools are not too happy about this but Labour have to get the money from somewhere.

He talks a lot about oracy skills and he has pledged to improve children's speaking skills, as part of a drive to break down class barriers to opportunity. He said it is "short-sighted" not to teach children how to "express" themselves. An "inability to articulate your thoughts fluently is a key barrier to getting on and thriving in life".

"It's key to doing well in a job interview, persuading a business to give you a refund, telling your friend something awkward. Oracy is a skill that can and must be taught."

This is so true. You can judge people by how they look but the minute they open their mouth to speak your impression can change instantly.

He also promised to give vocational and academic learning equal status and he will stress the need to tackle child poverty, with specialists on the issue being sent into the education system. He said more children should study sport or a creative arts subject until they are 16, as well as a focus on digital skills.

"For our children to succeed, they need a grounding in both. They need skills and knowledge, practical problem-solving and academic rigour," he said.

"But now - as the future rushes towards us, we also need a greater emphasis on creativity, on resilience, on emotional intelligence and the ability to adapt."

But just listen to this. It is music to my ears.

When he was young Sir Keir played the piano, the recorder, the violin and the flute. He became a junior scholar at the London Guildhall School of Music

In a speech in 2021, Sir Keir called for "every child" to have the chance to play a musical instrument in schools across the country.

He has spoken to Classic FM Requests presenter, Anne-Marie Minhall, to Sir Simon Rattle and to Andrew Lloyd Webber about the disappearance of music from many state schools.

"Music should, in my view be in every school, not just some."

He added that, alongside the joy music can bring, it also helps young people to develop skills like leadership, communication and team-work that they will eventually take into the workplace.

"I think that we have lost sight of the value of music in learning, and I'm determined to put that back in," he said.

Mozart was his favourite composer to play on the flute when he was a student.

"There's a special role for flute in Mozart," Sir Keir explained, describing the classical composer's writing for the instrument as "so profound".

He listens to the second movement of Beethoven's Emperor Piano Concerto to help him relax.

Well this is amazing. Mozart? Beethoven? I have never heard these names pass the lips of any other politician.

For me and for many others like me who love classical music and especially Mozart and Beethoven he has got my vote for that alone.

****

As we listen to the King's Speech today (November 7th) we hear Rishi Sunak wanting to make Britain a better place for everyone. It is completely nonsensical. They have had 13 years in which Britain has become poorer and poorer. Just some banal bills about crime and punishment, about gas and oil licences, about smoking and vaping.

About Education, Children's Care Homes, Children and Health, Children and Prison, Child Refugees, Poverty, the Arts and Music, or the Early Years...........................

NOTHING.

There is talk about the possibility of a General Election in either May or June 2024 although Sunak has hinted at October or even November. But it is only when this Labour government gets into power that our children and young people will have any hope for their future. Of course it will all take time and we wait to see exactly how this will all be achieved. But be assured, I will be watching very closely!

****

And at the moment the future is looking particularly grim. It is the week beginning the 13th of November 2023.

On **Monday** Suella Braverman was sacked as Home Secretary, by Rishi Sunak.

On **Tuesday** James Cleverly left his ministry of the Foreign Office and became the new Home Secretary. David Cameron the former prime minister became the new Foreign Secretary. How can this be exactly, I hear you asking, because he is not an MP? He was made a Life Peer so will sit in the House of Lords. He won't be able to speak in the Commons so everyday business will be delegated to whoever is seen as Cameron's number two – currently this would be Andrew Mitchell, the international development minister.

Then we hear that Esther McVey has been appointed Minister for Common Sense. Oh my goodness, you couldn't make it up.

On **Wednesday** the UK Supreme Court ruled that the Rwanda plan was unlawful. Rwanda was not a safe place.

On **Thursday** Sunak said he would not be ruled by foreign courts (!) and he would form a treaty which would say that Rwanda **is** a safe country.

Lord Sumption, a former justice of the Supreme Court, said that was "constitutionally extraordinary." I think that is posh speak for "absolutely anarchical suicide."

On **Friday** we hear further details of the Chancellor's autumn statement. We already know that he is going to cut benefits from people with long term illness and the disabled if they refuse to look for work. But today we hear that that will also mean they will not be eligible for free prescriptions or dental treatment, or help with public transport costs or any legal advice so keeping them in severe ill-health for even longer.

The face of compassionate Conservatism. Or have I said that before?

****

Today (22nd November) we hear the Chancellor's Autumn budget.

Well he obviously thought it was all marvellous and we should be very grateful for everything because as I watched him he was very bouncy and chirpy. But already there is a huge backlash from those who have studied it carefully. What I see is that there is nothing for education or the NHS and there is to be a cash freeze to investment spending. I can't believe this. This will mean our buildings will continue to crumble around our ears and our public services will continue to fall apart.

Then I receive an email from 'openDemocracy' with a critique written by the renowned economist **Ann Pettifor.**

It is damning but very explanatory. She headlines it as another autumn statement without any hope of an economic revival.

As she explains so clearly, in days gone by free education was provided in England and Wales because it was understood that for the functioning of society and the economy we needed educated and skilled workers. Gradually this was enhanced to include good health, housing and transport. But after 2010 all that stopped. We have seen and experienced a massive decline in all public services with the recent Conservative governments and our economy has suffered accordingly. And according to the TUC real terms pay remains 2.9% lower than in 2008.

"Fundamentally," she says, "we need to restructure our economy – away from a dependence on dirty fuels and physical infrastructure. We can do this by investing in social infrastructure (schools, universities, hospitals, community housing) as well as services like music, art, social and childcare – along with retrofitting and building green social homes, and upskilling and re-skilling our workforce. Such investment will generate savings and tax revenues, balance the budget, and get us on track to meet our climate commitments."

Oh my goodness what incredible common sense. And didn't **Boris Johnson**, in his conference speech in October 2021, say that he was aiming to turn the UK into a **"high wage, high skilled, high productivity economy"?** Well that is a rhetorical question because he did say that and I quote him on page 11 of **"Behind the Headlines"**. So here we are, over two years later, and still in an absolute bind.

And as Torsten Bell, the chief executive at the 'Resolution Foundation' think tank, said: "The truth is taxes are up not down. Today's cuts are dwarfed by tax rises already underway."

Nothing has improved and young people especially, will feel forgotten. The future is theirs and it is up to all of us to make the right choices in order to atone for the past. It will be a long journey and Labour will very likely make mistakes along the way.

But they need their chance and we can hold them to account by all these promises which I highlight in this chapter!

As we enter 2024 which is almost certain to be an election year, and as I bring this book to a close, I ask you to please, please stand up and speak out for our children. I believe that nothing is more important than that. And to all the charities looking after our children .... I salute you.

****

*"Children are the living messages
we send to a time we will not see."*

Neil Postman (American author.)

****

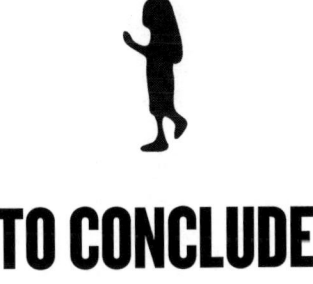

TO CONCLUDE

I believe that we need to listen carefully to the wise men and women who lived many years ago. Take note of what they say and although I have said I despair many times throughout this book, we must have hope in our hearts that there is a better future for our children and our grand-children.

****

"If we were logical, the future would be bleak, indeed. But we are more than logical. We are human beings, and we have faith, and we have hope, and we can work."

Jacques Yves Cousteau

****

"Perhaps the best hope for the future of mankind is that ways will be found of increasing the scope and intensity of sympathy"

Bertrand Russell

****

"Do your little bit of good where you are; it's those little bits of good put together that overwhelm the world."

Desmond Tutu

****

"The rich nations must use their vast resources of wealth to develop the underdeveloped, school the unschooled, and feed the unfed. Ultimately a great nation is a compassionate nation. No individual or nation can be great if it does not have a concern for 'the least of these.'"

Martin Luther King Jr.

****

But I conclude by quoting the greatest and most influential scientist of all time, a man of genius and a deep-thinking philosopher, who believed that imagination is more important than knowledge and he sends us this message for our children. This is my favourite quote of them all.

"If you want your children to be intelligent, read them fairy tales. If you want them to be more intelligent, read them more fairy tales."

Albert Einstein

****

Please listen to our children. Keep them safe. Support them. Understand their needs.

****

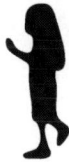

CHARITIES MENTIONED IN THIS BOOK

- **Save the Children.** Working alongside children in 115 countries, including the UK. P.1

- **Just for Kids Law**. Working with and for young people to ensure their legal rights are respected and promoted and their voices heard and valued. P.3

- **Banardos**. This is a children's charity that protects, supports and nurtures children across the UK who need help. It is the UK's largest children's charity, in terms of charitable expenditure. P.5

- **The Joseph Rowntree Foundation**. A responsive grant- making Quaker Trust. P. 6

- **National Youth Agency.** Transform the lives of young people in England and beyond through the power of youth work. P.17

- **UK Youth**. Focused on unlocking youth work as the catalyst of change that is needed now more than ever. P. 18

- **Ben Kinsella Trust**. Campaigns for action and justice for those affected by knife crime and educates young people so that they can make positive choices to stay safe. P. 21

- **Children's Society**. Work with young people who have suffered years of abuse, who have run away from home or are struggling with mental health issues. They look out for young carers and those who are at risk of being groomed by criminal groups. They help refugees who have no one else to turn to in this country. P.22

- **London Youth.** Work for children to have fun with their friends, to be healthy and creative, to make positive change in their communities, and to shape the kind of city they want for the future. P.23

- **Swim England.** From learners to teachers, athletes to coaches, we support people to achieve their best in the water. P.27

- **Education Support.** A UK charity dedicated to supporting the mental health and wellbeing of teachers and education staff in schools, colleges and universities. P.34

- **Chefs in Schools.** Have a proven model that embeds food education at the heart of a school and enables kitchen teams to serve up meals made from scratch with love, packed with fresh ingredients. P.35

- **School Food Matters.** Provide fully funded food education programmes to schools. P.36

- **NSPCC.** Working tirelessly to prevent child abuse. P.42

- **National Literacy Trust.** Developing the most effective tools and techniques for teachers and educators to support literacy, providing both resources and programmes designed to engage and inspire children, especially those who have had a tough start in life. P.47

- **Go Beyond.** A small charity that offers fun and enriching breaks packed with activities and adventures for children who care for their ill parents or have other challenges. P.69

- **Magic Breakfast**. Delivers free breakfasts to school children facing hunger everyday. P70

- **Howard League**. The oldest prison charity working for less crime, safer communities and fewer people in prison. P.90

- **Article 39.** A small, independent charity which fights for the rights of children living in state and privately-run institutions (boarding and residential schools, children's homes, immigration detention, mental health inpatient units, prisons and supported accommodation) in England. Their **name is taken from Article 39 of the** United Nations Convention on the Rights of the Child, **which grants every child who has been abused or suffered other rights violations the right to recover in environments where their health, self-respect and dignity are nurtured. P.92**

- **Asthma +Lung UK.** The UK's lung charity fighting for your right to breathe. P.101

- **Ash.** Is an independent public health charity set up by the Royal College of Physicians to end the harm caused by tobacco. P.102

- **Patient Safety Learning-the Hub.** A charity improving patient safety. P108

- **First Steps Nutrition.** Endeavour to fill practical and policy-relevant information gaps and provide resources for health workers supporting eating well from pre-conception to five years. P.124

- **Together for Short Lives.** Providing support, care and funding for children and young people needing palliative care. P.127

- **Beat.** A charity that provides support, information and resources for people affected by eating disorders and their carers. P.129

- **Children Heard and Seen.** A **charity** which provides support and interventions for **children** with a parent in prison. P.131

- **The Nuffield Trust.** A charity think tank which aims to influence policy and practice through generating and synthesising information on health and social care to facilitate both better policy and better practice. P.139

- **The Childhood Trust.** Dedicated to alleviating the impact of poverty on children and young people living in London. P.150

- **The Child Poverty Action Group.** Works on behalf of the more than one in four children in the UK growing up in poverty. P 155

- **Liberty.** Challenges injustice, defends freedom and campaigns to make sure everyone in the UK is treated fairly. They stand up to power. P.153

- **The Trussell Trust.** Support more than 1,300 food bank centres in a nationwide network of food banks and provide emergency food and support to people locked in poverty. They campaign for change to end the need for food banks in the UK. P.159

- **Shelter.** Exist to defend the right to a safe home. Because home is everything. P.168

- **Pregnant then Screwed.** Seeks to protect, support and promote the rights of pregnant women and mothers. P.173

- **Multibank.** Comic Relief and Amazon have launched a dedicated Multibank Fund to help finance the expansion of the Multibank initiative, co-founded by Amazon and former Prime Minister Gordon Brown in 2022. P.174

- **Zarach.** Provides beds and bedding to children in poverty. P.174

- **The Refugee Council.** The only national service offering support to all unaccompanied refugee children who arrive alone seeking safety in England. P.177

- **Human For Rights Network.** Documents rights violations against refugees, asylum seekers and migrants throughout Europe. P.180

- **The Sutton Trust.** An educational charity in the United Kingdom which aims to improve social mobility and address educational disadvantage. P.190

- **Speech and Language UK.** Give children and young people the skills they need so they aren't left behind, waiting to be understood. P.191

- **West London Zone.** Building trusted relationships, providing specialist support and joininjoining up each child's support system, including families, schools and local organorganisations, to deliver a personalised 2-year support plan for each child. P.205

- **Ambition Institute.** Provides the highest quality professional development, based on the most rigorous evidence of what really works, for teachers and school leaders at every stage in their their career. P.206

- **Feed.** Their mission is to change the face of infant feeding support in the UK. They support the Mum, not the method. P.210

****

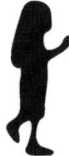

REPORTS REFERRED
TO IN THIS BOOK

- Save the Children Covid-19 Inquiry report 'What About The Children?' in partnership with the Children's Rights Alliance for England and Just for Kids Law, and backed by former Children's Commissioner Anne Longfield. Sept. 2023. P.3

- Office for National Statistics: Crime in England and Wales 2023. P.25

- The Youth Endowment Fund: Children, violence and vulnerability. 2023. P.25

- Swim England's Value of Swimming report. 2023 P.27

- Primary School Library Alliance report (in conjunction with the National Literacy Trust) October 2021. P.47

- Institute on Fiscal Studies: Education spending in England. 2023 Annual report. P.51

- National Student Accommodation Survey. P.56

- National Foundation for Educational research: Teacher Labour Market in England. 2023. P.60

- Public First Report. December 2023. (commissioned by the Laidlaw Foundation) P.61

- The Times Education Commission report. 2022. P.63

- House of Commons Committee report: Education Recovery in Schools in England. June 2023. P.65

- The Committee of Public Accounts: The condition of school buildings.November 2023. P.72

- Healing Justice, London. P.76

- The Equality & Human Rights Monitor Report. UK Parliament. 2023 P. 76

- Competition and Market Authority. P.83

- Children's Commission on Private Provision in Children's Social Care.November 2020. P.85

- Child Safeguarding Practice Review Panel report. GOV UK P.88

- The Institute for Government's Year in Review. December 2023. P.94

- The Royal College of Paediatrics: State of Child Health. 2020 P. 97

- The Ockenden Report. P.114

- NHS Ombudsman report P.118

- Care Quality Commissions Annual report 2023 P.118

- Save the Children Annual Report 2018 P.119

- Mothers and Babies: Reducing Risk through Audits and Confidential Enquiries across the UK. P.122

- The Right to Family Life: children whose mothers are in prison. A House of Commons Committee report.2019. P.135

- HM Chief Inspector of Prisons, England and Wales Annual Report 2022-2023. P.141

- The London Child Poverty Report. 2021. The Childhood Trust. P.151

- Destitution in the UK. 2023 Joseph Rowntree Foundation. P.157

- Hunger in the UK. The Trussell Trust. June 2023 P.159

- Ministry of Housing Committee and Local Government annual report. P. 170

- International Covenant on Economics, Social and Cultural Rights. P.172

- Pregnant then Screwed report March 2023. P.173

- Refugee Council. P.177

- Humans for Rights Network. P.180

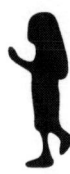

ACKNOWLEDGEMENTS

I want to say a huge thank you once again to all journalists and columnists everywhere. The accurate and fearless reporting of news is more important than ever before.

My thanks go to:

The Times	Sky News
The Sunday Times	LBC
The Financial Times	Channel 4
The Sun	The Good Law Project
The Guardian	openDemocracy
The I	38 Degrees
The Observer	Care4Calais
The Independent	Politics home
The Evening Standard	Twitter
The Mirror	HuffPost
The Daily Mail	Left Foot Forward
The Daily Telegraph	The Canary
The Express	HOPE not Hate

Many, many people, charities and protest groups have been credited throughout this text and if I have left anyone out I apologise. But without all of you this book could never have been written.

ABOUT THE AUTHOR

Sue Wood was born and brought up in a medical family in Coventry. She was educated in Leamington Spa and Maria Grey Froebel College in Twickenham. She worked as a Primary school teacher in Coventry and Cambridge and then took a break from teaching and worked as Director of Public Relations at Coventry Cathedral. After her wedding there she moved with her husband first to Abu Dhabi and then to Aberdeen. She is now settled in Hertfordshire with her husband and has two children and two grand-children.

She returned to teaching, first in Bushey and then in Elstree. On retiring she became a volunteer Speaker for Save the Children. She has always been concerned about those whom she feels are being treated unjustly and has been a member of the Howard League for Penal Reform for over 30 years.

She started writing at the age of 10 when her American aunt gave her a 5 year diary, and she has written many books for family and friends. Her first three published books for the general public are:-

Beneath the Bluster. A Diary of Despair. Ignorance, Incompetence, Confusion and Lies. The Conservative Government 2019-2021

Behind the Headlines. A Parallel Universe. Arrogance, Corruption, Dither and Delay. The Conservative Government 2021-2022.

Britain Betrayed. Slash and Burn. Delusional, Dysfunctional, Dishonest, and Degenerate. The Conservative Government 2022-2023.

She has always been interested in news and politics, and these three books together cover the most shameful period in the history of the UK.